Therapy for Genitourinary Cancer

Cancer Treatment and Research

WILLIAM L. MCGUIRE, *series editor*

Livingston, R.B. (ed): Lung Cancer 1. 1981. ISBN 90-247-2394-9
Humphrey G.B., Dehner L.P., Grindey G.B., Acton R.T. (eds): Pediatric Oncology 1. ISBN 90-274-2408-2
DeCosse J.J., Sherlock P. (eds): Gastrointestinal Cancer 1. 1981. ISBN 90-247-2461-9
Bennett J.M. (ed): Lymphomas 1, including Hodgkin's Disease. 1981. ISBN 90-247-2479-1
Bloomfield C.D. (ed): Adult Leukemias 1. 1982. ISBN 90-247-2478-3
Paulson D.F. (ed): Genitourinary Cancer 1. 1982. ISBN 90-247-2480-5
Muggia F.M. (ed): Cancer Chemotherapy 1. 1983. ISBN 90-247-2713-8
Humphrey G.B., Grindey G.B. (eds): Pancreatic Tumors in Children. 1982. ISBN 90-247-2702-2
Costanzi J.J. (ed): Malignant Melanoma 1. 1983. ISBN 90-247-2706-5
Griffiths C.T., Fuller A.F. (eds): Gynecologic Oncology. 1983. ISBN 0-89838-555-5
Greco A.F. (ed): Biology and Management of Lung Cancer. 1983. ISBN 0-89838-554-7
Walker M.D. (ed): Oncology of the Nervous System. 1983. ISBN 0-89838-567-9
Higby D.J. (ed): Supportive Care in Cancer Therapy. 1983. ISBN 0-89838-569-5
Herberman R.B. (ed): Basic and Clinical Tumor Immunology. 1983. ISBN 0-89838-579-2
Baker L.H. (ed): Soft Tissue Sarcomas. 1983. ISBN 0-89838-584-9
Bennett J.M. (ed): Controversies in the Management of Lymphomas. 1983. ISBN 0-89838-586-5
Humphrey G.B., Grindey G.B. (eds): Adrenal and Endocrine Tumors in Children. 1983. ISBN 0-89838-590-3
DeCosse J.J., Sherlock P. (eds): Clinical Management of Gastrointestinal Cancer. 1984. ISBN 0-89838-601-2
Catalona W.J., Ratliff T.L. (eds): Urologic Oncology. 1984. ISBN 0-89838-628-4
Santen R.J., Manni A. (eds): Diagnosis and Management of Endocrine-Related Tumors. 1984. ISBN 0-89838-636-5
Costanzi J.J. (ed): Clinical Management of Malignant Melanoma. 1984. ISBN 0-89838-656-X
Wolf G.T. (ed): Head and Neck Oncology. 1984. ISBN 0-89838-657-8
Alberts D.S., Surwit E.A. (eds): Ovarian Cancer. 1985. ISBN 0-89838-676-4
Muggia F.M. (ed): Experimental and Clinical Progress in Cancer Chemotherapy. 1985. ISBN 0-89838-679-9
Higby D.J. (ed): Issues in Supportive Care of Cancer Patients. 1986. ISBN 0-89838-816-3
Surwit E.A., Alberts D.S. (eds): Cervix Cancer. 1987. ISBN 0-89838-822-8
Jacobs C. (ed): Cancers of the Head and Neck. 1987. ISBN 0-89838-825-2
MacDonald J.S. (ed): Gastrointestinal Oncology. 1987. ISBN 0-89838-829-5
Ratliff T.L., Catalona W.J. (eds): Genitourinary Cancer. 1987. ISBN 0-89838-830-9
Nathanson L. (ed): Basic and Clinical Aspects of Malignant Melanoma. 1987. ISBN 0-89838-856-2
Muggia F.M. (ed): Concepts, Clinical Developments, and Therapeutic Advances in Cancer Chemotherapy. 1987. ISBN 0-89838-879-5
Frankel A.E. (ed): Immunotoxins. 1988. ISBN 0-89838-984-4
Bennett J.M., Foon K.A. (eds): Immunologic Approaches to the Classification and Management of Lymphomas and Leukemias. 1988. ISBN 0-89838-355-2
Osborne C.K. (ed): Endocrine Therapies in Breast and Prostate Cancer. 1988. ISBN 0-89838-365-X
Lippman M.E., Dickson R. (eds): Breast Cancer: Cellular and Molecular Biology. 1988. ISBN 0-89838-368-4
Kamps W.A., Humphrey G.B., Poppema S. (eds): Hodgkin's Disease in Children: Controversies and Current Practice. 1988. ISBN 0-89838-372-2
Muggia F.M. (ed): Cancer Chemotherapy: Concepts, Clinical Investigations and Therapeutic Advances. 1988. ISBN 0-89838-381-1
Nathanson L. (ed): Malignant Melanoma: Biology, Diagnosis, and Therapy. 1988. ISBN 0-89838-384-6
Pinedo H.M., Verweij J. (eds): Treatment of Soft Tissue Sarcomas. 1989. ISBN 0-89838-391-9
Hansen H.H. (ed): Basic and Clinical Concepts of Lung Cancer. 1989. ISBN 0-7923-0153-6
Lepor H., Ratliff T.L. (eds): Urologic Oncology. 1989. ISBN 0-7923-0161-7
Benz C., Liu E. (eds): Oncogenes. 1989. ISBN 0-7923-0237-0
Ozols R.F. (ed): Drug Resistance in Cancer Therapy. 1989. ISBN 0-7923-0244-3
Surwit E.A., Alberts D.S. (eds): Endometrial Cancer. 1989. ISBN 0-7923-0286-9
Champlin R. (ed): Bone Marrow Transplantation. 1990. ISBN 0-7923-0612-0
Goldenberg D. (ed): Cancer Imaging with Radiolabeled Antibodies. 1990. ISBN 0-7923-0631-7
Jacobs C. (ed): Carcinomas of the Head and Neck. 1990. ISBN 0-7923-0668-6
Lippman M.E., Dickson R. (eds): Regulatory Mechanisms in Breast Cancer: Advances in Cellular and Molecular Biology of Breast Cancer. 1990. ISBN 0-7923-0868-9
Nathanson, L. (ed): Maligant Melanoma: Genetics, Growth Factors, Metastases, and Antigens. 1991. ISBN 0-7923-0895-6
Sugarbaker, P.H. (ed): Management of Gastric Cancer. 1991. ISBN 0-7923-1102-7
Pinedo H.M., Verweij J., Suit, H.D., (eds): Soft Tissue Sarcomas: New Developments in the Multidisciplinary Approach to Treatment. ISBN 0-7923-1139-6
Ozols, R.F., (ed): Molecular and Clinical Advances in Anticancer Drug Resistance. 1991. ISBN 0-7923-1212-0
Muggia, F.M. (ed): New Drugs, Concepts and Results in Cancer Chemotherapy 1991.

Therapy for Genitourinary Cancer

edited by

Herbert Lepor
and
Russell K. Lawson
The Medical College of Wisconsin
Froedtert Memorial Lutheran Hospital
Milwaukee, Wisconsin USA

1992 **KLUWER ACADEMIC PUBLISHERS**
BOSTON / DORDRECHT / LONDON

Distributors

for North America: Kluwer Academic Publishers, 101 Philip Drive, Assinippi Park, Norwell, Massachusetts 02061 USA
for all other countries: Kluwer Academic Publishers Group, Distribution Centre, Post Office Box 322, 3300 AH Dordrecht, The Netherlands

Cancer Treatment and Research is indexed in the National Library of Medicine MEDLARS system.

Library of Congress Cataloging-in-Publication Data

Therapy for genitourinary cancer/edited by Herbert Lepor and Russell K. Lawson.
p. cm. — (Cancer treatment and research; v. 59)
Includes bibliographical references and index.
ISBN 0-7923-1412-3
1. Genitourinary organs—Cancer—Treatment. I. Lepor, Herbert. II. Lawson, Russell K. III. Series.
[DNLM: 1. Urogenital Neoplasms—therapy. W1 CA693 v. 59/WJ 160 T3988]
RC280.G4T55 1992
616.99'4606—dc20
DNLM/DLC
for Library of Congress 91-20877
CIP

Copyright

PRINTED IN THE UNITED STATES OF AMERICA.

Printed on acid-free paper.

Table of Contents

Foreword to the Series vii
Preface ix
List of Contributors xi

1. Genitourinary rhabdomyosarcoma in childhood: Current treatment alternatives and controversies in management 1
E. SHAPIRO and D. STROTHER

2. Renal-sparing surgery for renal and transitional cell carcinoma 19
R.K. LAWSON

3. A comparison of the treatment of metastatic prostate cancer by testicular ablation or total androgen blockade 29
THE CANADIAN ANANDRON STUDY GROUP

4. The role of radiotherapy following radical prostatectomy 41
M.K. BRAWER

5. Nuclear DNA ploidy and prostate cancer 53
L.M. RAINWATER and H. ZINCKE

6. Brachytherapy of localized penile carcinoma 65
R.W. BYHARDT and J.F. WILSON

7. Malignancy associated with urinary tract reconstruction using enteric segments 75
J.R. SPENCER and R.B. FILMER

8. Evolving concepts in surgical management of testis cancer 89
J.P. DONOHUE, R. BIHRLE, and R.S. FOSTER

9. Neoadjuvant chemotherapy and partial cystectomy for invasive bladder cancer 99
H.W. HERR and H.I. SCHER

10. Tumor necrosis factor and chemotherapeutic drugs targeted at DNA topoisomerase II for the treatment of genitourinary malignancies 105
R.B. ALEXANDER

11. Cell motility as an index of metastatic ability in prostate cancers: Results with an animal model and with human cancer cells 121
A.W. PARTIN, J.L. MOHLER, and D.S. COFFEY

12. Suramin as an archetypical compound in the development of growth factor antagonists for inhibition of genitourinary tumors 131
H.I. SCHER and W.D.W. HESTON

Index 153

Cancer Treatment and Research Foreword

Where do you begin to look for a recent, authoritative article on the diagnosis or management of a particular malignancy? The few general oncology textbooks are generally out of date. Single papers in specialized journals are informative but seldom comprehensive; these are more often preliminary reports on a very limited number of patients. Certain general journals frequently publish good in-depth reviews of cancer topics, and published symposium lectures are often the best overviews available. Unfortunately, these reviews and supplements appear sporadically, and the reader can never be sure when a topic of special interest will be covered.

Cancer Treatment and Research is a series of authoritative volumes that aim to meet this need. It is an attempt to establish a critical mass of oncology literature covering virtually all oncology topics, revised frequently to keep the coverage up to date, and easily available on a single library shelf or by a single personal subscription.

We have approached the problem in the following fashion: first, by dividing the oncology literature into specific subdivisions, such as lung cancer, genitourinary cancer, pediatric oncology, etc.; and second, by asking eminent authorities in each of these areas to edit a volume on the specific topic on an annual or biannual basis. Each topic and tumor type is covered in a volume appearing frequently and predictably, discussing current diagnosis, staging, markers, all forms of treatment modalities, basic biology, and more.

In *Cancer Treatment and Research*, we have an outstanding group of editors, each having made a major commitment to bring to this new series the very best literature in his or her field. Kluwer Academic Publishers has made an equally major commitment to the rapid publication of high-quality books and to worldwide distribution.

Where can you go to find quickly a recent authoritative article on any major oncology problem? We hope that *Cancer Treatment and Research* provides an answer.

William L. McGuire
Series Editor

Preface

The ultimate objective of therapy for genitourinary malignancies is cure without adversely affecting the quality of life. *Therapy for Genitourinary Cancer* addresses modifications of standard surgical procedures that purport to decrease the morbidity of therapy for testis cancer and renal cell carcinoma without compromising cure. In addition, the rationale for decreasing the extent of surgical extirpation for bladder cancer and rhabdomyosarcoma are summarized. The ability to limit the extent of therapy depends upon the ability to predict the metastatic potential of the primary tumor. The application of cell motility and DNA ploidy to predict the metastatic potential of prostate cancer are presented. Prostate cancer represents the second most common cause of cancer-related deaths among American males. Due to the realization that little progress has been made to enhance survival rates for prostate cancer, more aggressive treatment regimens are presently being advocated. The role of adjuvant radiotherapy following radical prostatectomy and complete androgen suppression for metastatic prostate cancer are reviewed. Chemotherapy for prostate cancer has proven to be disappointing. The preliminary experiences with suramin and the implications of combining tumor necrosis factor and chemotherapeutic drugs are presented. The use of bladder substitution with intestinal segments has enhanced the quality of life following pelvic extirpative surgery. The development of carcinoma in these intestinal bladders is discussed.

The contents of *Therapy for Genitourinary Cancer* reflects the commitment of clinicians and basic scientists to enhance the effectiveness of therapy for genitourinary malignancies. The editors are grateful for the scholarly manuscripts submitted by all of the contributors. Several of the diagnostic and treatment modalities for genitourinary malignancies presented in *Therapy for Genitourinary Cancer* are in their early stages of investigation. Hopefully, these innovative approaches to the treatment of genitourinary malignancy will gain clinical acceptance and improve our ability to cure these tumors.

HERBERT LEPOR
RUSSELL K. LAWSON
Editors

List of contributors

ALEXANDER, Richard B., Senior Investigator, Division of Urologic Oncology, Surgery Branch, National Cancer Institute, Bldg. 10, Room 2B56, Bethesda, MD 20892

BIHRLE, Richard, Associate Professor, Department of Urology, Indiana University School of Medicine, 926 W. Michigan Street, Indianapolis, IN 46202-5250

BRAWER, Michael K., Assistant Professor, Department of Urology, University of Washington, Seattle, WA 98195

BYHARDT, Roger W., Professor, Department of Radiation/Oncology, Medical College of Wisconsin, 8700 W. Wisconsin Avenue, Milwaukee, WI 53226

COFFEY, Donald S., Professor of Urology, Oncology and Pharmacology, The Johns Hopkins University School of Medicine, 600 North Wolfe Street, Marburg 134, Baltimore, MD 212015

DONOHUE, John P., Professor and Chairman, Indiana University School of Medicine, 926 W. Michigan Street, Indianapolis, IN 46202-5250

FILMER, R. Bruce, Division of Urology, Alfred I. Dupont Institute, Wilmington, DE 19850

FOSTER, Richard S., Assistant Professor, Department of Urology, Indiana University School of Medicine, 926 W. Michigan Street, Indianapolis, IN 46202-5250

HERR, Harry W., Professor, Department of Urology, Sloan Kettering Cancer Center, 1275 York Avenue, New York, NY 10021

HESTON, Warren W.D., Director, Urologic Oncology Research, Memorial Sloan Kettering Cancer Center, 1275 York Avenue, New York, NY 10021

LAWSON, Russell K., Professor and Chairman, Department of Urology, The Medical College of Wisconsin, 9200 W. Wisconsin Avenue, Milwaukee, WI 53226

PARTIN, Allen, W., Resident, Department of Urology, The Johns Hopkins University School of Medicine, 600 N. Wolfe Street, Marburg 134, Baltimore, MD 21205

RAINWATER, Leslie M., Senior Resident, Urology, Mayo Graduate School of Medicine, Rochester, MN 55905

SCHER, Howard I., Department of Medicine, Cornell University Medical College, 1275 York Avenue, New York, NY 10021

SHAPIRO, Ellen, Associate Professor of Surgery, Medical College of Wisconsin, 9200 W. Wisconsin Avenue, Milwaukee, WI 53226

SPENCER, Julia R., Assistant Professor of Surgery, Cornell University School of Medicine, 525 East 68th Street, New York, NY 10021

STROTHER, Douglas, Assistant Professor of Pediatrics, Medical College of Wisconsin, 9200 W. Wisconsin Avenue, Milwaukee, WI 53226

TRACHTENBERG, John, Associate Professor, Department of Surgery, University of Toronto, 101 College Street, Toronto, Ontario M5G 979, Canada

WILSON, J. Frank, Professor and Chairman, Department of Radiation/Oncology, Medical College of Wisconsin, 8700 W. Wisconsin Avenue, Milwaukee, WI 53226

ZINCKE, Horst, Professor of Urology, Mayo Medical School, Rochester, MN 55905

Therapy for Genitourinary Cancer

1. Genitourinary rhabdomyosarcoma in childhood: Current treatment alternatives and controversies in management

Ellen Shapiro and Douglas Strother

Rhabdomyosarcoma (RMS) is the most common soft-tissue sarcoma of childhood and accounts for 4–8% of all malignant disease in children less than 15 years of age. It constitutes 5–15% of all malignant solid tumors. Among solid tumors, it is exceeded in frequency only by brain neoplasms, neuroblastoma, and Wilm's tumor. Approximately 15–20% of RMS are genitourinary (GU) in origin and arise from the same embryonal mesenchyme that gives rise to striated skeletal muscle [1,2].

Treatment for GU RMS has evolved over the years and treating physicians have tried to maintain a balance between high survival rates and preservation of the genitourinary tract to ensure the quality of life. Prior to 1960, the treatment of GU RMS consisted of extirpative surgery and radiation, either alone or in combination. In 1959, one of the earliest reviews of bladder sarcomas in children reported 80 cases diagnosed after 1900 [3]. There were only six known survivors and the earliest disease-free survior was not reported until 1952 [4].

Significant advances have been made over the past two decades in understanding the biological activity of this tumor. The rationale for a multitherapeutic approach has come from the efforts of three cooperative cancer study groups. These groups combined their resources in 1972 to form the Intergroup Rhabdomyosarcoma Study (IRS). This multicenter effort has resulted in several clinical trials (IRS-I 1972–1978, IRS-II 1978–1984, IRS-III 1984–1988, and IRS-IV 1989–present). The evolution of our treatment approach to the patient with rhabdomyosarcoma is the result of the outcomes of these studies.

This chapter will review GU RMS, including those of the bladder, prostate, vagina, uterus, cervix, and vulva, and controversies in their management. Paratesticular RMS will be discussed separately at the end of this chapter.

Epidemiology

The estimated annual incidence of genitourinary rhabdomyosarcoma is 0.5–0.7 cases per one million children under age 15. The tumor occurs with

Lepor, H. and Lawson R.K., (eds.), Therapy for Genitourinary Cancer. *ISBN 0-7923-1412-3.*

a male predominance of 3:1 [5]. Rhabdomyosarcoma of urogenital origin occurs at two age peaks: the first, in children between 2 and 6 years, and the second, during adolescence between 15 and 19 years [6]. Rhabdomyosarcoma has been associated with several congenital disorders, including neurofibromatosis, Gorlin's basal-cell nevus syndrome, and the fetal alcohol syndrome [7]. There also appears to be a genetic component to this tumor. Li and Fraumeni have identified familial aggregations of rhabdomyosarcoma with other sarcomas, breast cancers, and brain tumors [8]. Other familial associations have been reported with an increased incidence in RMS in the siblings of children with CNS tumors and adrenal cortical carcinoma [7].

Research advances

Cytogenetics

Advances have been made in determining the cytogenetic features of this tumor. Douglass et al. identified a distinct chromosomal translocation t(2;13)(q35;q14) in a direct preparation of rhabdomyosarcoma involving cells that had metatasized to bone marrow and in human tumor xenografts [9]. This translocation appears to be specific for RMS and has been found in embryonal, undifferentiated, and alveolar subtypes. IRS-IV will prospectively assess the clinical significance of this translocation, since it has been found in tumors from patients with advanced or recurrent disease. Investigation of his translocation may be useful in identifying patients who present with more advanced disease at diagnosis and those with disease that is refractory to current treatment protocols [10].

Molecular studies

Using human RMS cell lines, intracellular peptides that modulate cell growth activity, including transforming growth factors, tumor cell inhibitory factors, and the transforming oncogene *N-ras*, have been identified [7]. Experiments using the implantation of human RMS xenograft lines into nude mice have been invaluable in determining the sensitivity and resistance mechanisms of various cytologic agents. For example, vincristine resistance may be associated with the production of tubulin with an altered binding affinity, which affects drug retention by tumor tissues [11]. Also, the activity of an enzyme important in DNA repair has been shown to be positively correlated with the sensitivity of cell lines to nitrosourea methyl-CCNU [7].

IRS-IV proposes to examine RMS tumor cells to detect alterations of specific cellular proto-oncogenes that may have prognostic and therapeutic importance. Roberts et al. examined DNA from patients of RMS for evidence of amplification of the *gli* gene [12]. A 30-fold amplification of *gli* and detectable levels of *gli* mRNA transcripts were identified in rhabdomyoblasts. Other investigators have documented *N-myc* gene amplification in RMS, which has been an important prognostic indicator in patients with neuroblastoma [13–15]. IRS-IV will also be investigating the occurrence of abnormalities of not only the *N-myc* gene, but also abnormalities of other cellular proto-oncogenes, such as *C-myc*, *L-myc*, *NEU*, and *EGFR* [10].

Flow cytometric studies

Flow cytometric determination of cellular DNA content can be used to predict the prognosis in some childhood cancers. The DNA ploidy values appear to have different clinical implication in different types of childhood tumors. In a study from the Mayo Clinic, six patients with embryonal RMS of the bladder and prostate had DNA aneuploid tumors [16]. At the time of diagnosis, one patient was stage I and five patients were stage III. All of these patients responded well to a combination of chemotherapy and surgery. In the IRS tumor samples submitted thus far, there has been a correlation between tetraploidy patterns with alveolar histology and intermediate hyperdiploidy with embryonal histology [10]. The prognostic significance of these findings will need to be determined.

Monoclonal antibody studies

Monoclonal antibodies reacting with skeletal muscle markers, such as desmin and a muscle-specific isotype of actin, have been useful in the diagnosis of poorly differentiated RMS. Antibody probes (4.2A8, 5.1H11, and 3.1G11) developed by Dr. Peter J. Houghton appear to recognize embryonal but not alveolar RMS [10]. These monoclonal antibody studies may be important not only as a diagnostic tool, but also as a potential immunotherapeutic modality.

Pathology

Rhabdomyosarcoma arises from primitive mesenchymal cells that exhibit varying degrees of differentiation towards skeletal muscle, smooth muscle, and connective tissue [2,17–19]. Rhabdomyosarcomas are highly malignant and spread by local invasion, as well as lymphatic and hematogenous routes. Lymphatic metastases occur in approximately 20% of genitourinary RMS and may be as high as 40% in the subset of paratesticular tumors [20]. The most common sites of hematogenous spread include lung, bone marrow, and liver, and are present in up to 40% of patients at the time of diagnosis [21–23].

The histologic classification of RMS reflects the wide range of mesenchymal differences that may occur. The three major subtypes are embryonal, alveolar, and pleomorphic [24]. Embryonal RMS accounts for 50–60% of childhood RMS. Morphologically, embryonal RMS resembles developing skeletal muscle, as seen in the 7- to 10-week fetus, and is composed primarily of spindle-shaped cells with a central nucleus and abundant eosinophilic cytoplasm [24,25]. Cross-striations are important for diagnosis but are seen in only 30% of these tumors. The term *sarcoma botryoides* refers to a polypoid form of embryonal RMS and grossly appears as a cluster of grapes projecting intraluminally into a hollow viscus, such as the bladder or vagina [26]. Alveolar RMS is the second most common histologic subtype, resembling skeletal muscle in the 10- to 21-week fetus [25]. It has a unique pattern that is reminiscent of pulmonary alveoli [24]. Alveolar RMS is seen in older children and young adults, and most commonly accounts for extremity or perineal sites. It metastasizes to lymph nodes and has a poorer prognosis than embryonal RMS. The pleomorphic type of RMS is rarely seen in children and is most common in extremity and truncal tumors.

The IRS has further classified these tumors into *favorable* and *unfavorable* categories [27]. The unfavorable histologic types include 1) anaplastic RMS (enlarged bizarre mitotic figures and diffuse nuclear hyperchromatism with pleomorphism), 2) monomorphous round-cell RMS (marked uniformity in size and cytologic characteristics of the total tumor cell population), and 3) alveolar tumors. All other gross or cellular features are categorized as favorable.

Clinical presentation

Bladder rhabdomyosarcoma

Tumors originating in the submucosa or superficial layers of the trigone often present with bladder outlet obstruction [5,28,29]. This may lead to urinary retention, incontinence, and infection. Gross hematuria and passage of tissue fragments may occur when the tumor disrupts the overlying bladder mucosa. The tumor usually occurs in a distinctive botryoides form and often enlarges into a palpable suprapubic mass. It may extend into the membranous urethra in the male. In the female, the mass may expand along the entire length of the female urethra and present as a prolapsing mass [22]. Bladder RMS is more commonly seen in males (2:1), and patients are usually younger than 5 years of age [5]. The tumor may invade locally into the prostate, vulva, and vagina, and it is local extension that is the most common cause of treatment failures.

Prostatic rhabdomyosarcoma

Prostatic RMS tends to present as a solid mass, rather than in the botryoides form. It is often difficult to distinguish if the tumor arose from the prostate or from the bladder neck and trigone region. Local extension into the bladder neck and posterior urethra results in bladder outlet obstruction and a palpable bladder on physical examination. Expansile growth posteriorly causes a mass effect, with the tumor easily palpable on rectal exam. Local infiltration of the rectal wall leads to constipation as the presenting symptom. The median age for males with prostatic RMS is 3.5 years [5,28,29].

In a review of the occurrence of lymphatic metastases in childhood RMS, the IRS found nodal metastases to be greatest for primary prostate RMS (41%) [30]. Lymphatic involvement was also significant for paratesticular tumors (26%) and for genitourinary sites in general (24%), compared to only 14% for all RMS. Involvement of the lymph nodes was positively correlated with tumor size.

Female genital tract rhabdomyosarcoma

Primary vaginal rhabdomyosarcoma is the most common tumor of the female genital tract in children [31]. The mean age for vaginal RMS is younger than 2 years, while patients with uterine sarcoma present during adolescence. Vulvar lesions occur in a wide age spectrum (1–19 years). Vaginal tumors usually occur on the anterior vaginal wall adjacent to the cervix, but may also arise from other regions of the vagina. Patients present with hemorrhagic vaginal discharge or with vaginal extrusion of tumor fragments. Vaginal tumors may present with symptoms of urethral obstruction or a palpable abdominal mass. Local infiltration into the bladder wall is less common. The rectovaginal septum acts as a barrier, protecting the rectal wall from local infiltration.

Uterine RMS presents as a mass with a single large polyp proturding from the cervix or with intramural involvement of the cervix and/or body of the uterus [31]. Vulvar tumors present with a palpable mass involving the labia and are commonly mistaken for Bartholin's gland infections.

Radiographic evaluation

Ultrasound is usually the initial imaging modality for the evaluation of an infant presenting with a palpable abdominal mass [32]. A lobulated soft tissue mass within, displacing, or deforming the bladder suggests the diagnosis of pelvic RMS. The tumor may be totally or partially fixed to the pelvic floor. Usually RMS shows homogeneous echogenicity with an echotexture similar to that of muscle. However, areas of reduced echogenicity may be identified. The appearance may simulate a pelvic abscess. The regional and retroperitoneal nodes may be enlarged. Due to the small size of the bony pelvis in infants and young children, some degree of urinary tract obstruction is usually present.

In the past, intravenous pyelography (IVP) was the primary diagnostic imaging modality revealing various degrees of ureteropyelocaliectasis [28,32].

The cystogram phase often demonstrated the characteristic negative filling defect within the bladder when the bladder neck and trigone were the regions of origin. In prostatic RMS, the IVP demonstrates elevation of the bladder base, and a voiding cystourethrogram may demonstrate distortion and elongation of the prostatic urethra.

A suspected pelvic mass is currently evaluated with computed tomography (CT) using oral, rectal, and intravenous contrast [32]. The bladder must be filled to detect infiltration of the bladder wall. Pelvic RMS may be isodense with muscle or show lower attenuation. Focal areas of reduced density within the tumor are generally due to hemorrhage or necrosis. A bladder neck/trigone RMS may be difficult to differentiate on CT scan from tumors arising from the adjacent prostate gland. The CT findings in prostatic tumors include an enlarged homogeneous mass with invasion of the perirectal fat. Thickening of the levator ani muscle may be demonstrated, as well as tumor invasion into muscle and bone through the ischiorectal fossa and the sciatic and obturator foramen.

Magnetic resonance imaging (MRI) has offered a new potential for staging of bladder tumors [33]. MRI has better contrast resolution and comparable spatial resolution than CT. The ability of MRI to obtain sagittal and coronal sections is of great advantage in visualizing tumors of the bladder neck and dome. Extension of the neoplasm to the prostate and seminal vesicles can also be seen on MRI. Local extension of tumor can also be better appreciated using this imaging modality.

Diagnosis

Bladder RMS is diagnosed with cystoscopy and biopsy [29]. When obtaining a biopsy with a pediatric resectoscope, the use of the resectoscope loop electrode may result in excessive coagulation, making histologic interpretation difficult. The cold-cup biopsy forceps is generally more satisfactory. These may be passed through a 13-French resectoscope. The 10-French resectoscope can be used with a Collings knife electrode to remove a polypoid specimen by cutting through its base. In patients with prostatic involvement, tissue diagnosis is made by a transurethral biopsy. Perineal or extraperitoneal suprapubic biopsy may be performed with a Vim-Silverman or Tru-Cut needle. A laparotomy is rarely required in order to obtain tumor to establish a diagnosis. In patients with vaginal RMS, an endoscopic biopsy is performed. Local, gross, or partial tumor excision may be performed at the time of biopsy. Cystoscopy at the time of biopsy will determine extrinsic distortion or tumor infiltration of the bladder wall. Diagnosis of uterine sarcomas is commonly made by transvaginal biopsy aided by cervical dilatation and curettage. Patients presenting with vulvar lesions undergo incisional or excisional biopsy, or wide local excision if a frozen-section diagnosis can be made [31].

Table 1. Intergroup rhabdomyosarcoma study staging

Group I	Localized disease completely resected; regional nodes not involved A. Confined to muscle or organ of origin B. Contiguous involvement with infiltration outside the muscle or organ or origin, as through fascial planes
Group II	Regional disease A. Grossly resected tumor with microscopic residual disease; no evidence of gross residual tumor; no clinical or microscopic evidence of regional node involvement B. Regional disease, completely resected (regional nodes involved or extension of tumor into an adjacent organ; no microscopic residual disease) C. Regional disease with involved nodes, grossly resected, but with evidence of microscopic residual disease
Group III	Incomplete resection or biopsy with gross residual disease
Group IV	Distant metastatic disease present at onset

Tumor staging

Staging for RMS is dependent on the resectability of the primary tumor and nodal involvement. The IRS clinical grouping classification was proposed in 1977 and is presented in Table 1 [23,24]. A metastatic evaluation, including lung and abdominal CT and bone marrow aspiration, will evaluate the most common regions for lymphatic and hematogenous spread. Also, a bone survey or radionuclide bone scan is indicated.

Treatment

Historical

Prior to the advent of chemotherapeutic agents, RMS of the bladder and prostate was treated with surgery, including anterior or total pelvic exenteration. Rhabdomyosarcoma of the female genital tract was managed with radical hysterectomy and excision of the vaginal cuff. Local excision or segmental resection resulted in uniformly high pelvic recurrence rates and poor survival due to metastatic disease. When wide surgical excision was used as the single therapeutic modality, long-term survival for localized bladder and prostate RMS was 73%, while survival with vaginal tumors was only 40% [35].

Radiation therapy began to emerge when the 1950 report by Stobbe and Dargeon noted that some RMS were radiosensitive [36]. Single-agent chemotherapy, and subsequently a multiagent approach, were employed to first treat metastatic disease [35]. Synergy was soon recognized between actinomycin D (dactinomycin) and radiation therapy [37]. In 1961, Pinkel and Pickren suggested combining radical surgery with postoperative radiation and "prophylactic" chemotherapy following "complete" tumor resection [38]. In a study in which all children received radical surgery and postoperative radiation, those patients randomized to receive chemotherapy had an 85% 2-year relapse-free interval, while those not receiving chemotherapy had a 47% 2-year relapse-free interval.

Intergroup Rhabdomyosarcoma Study-I

Following this important pioneering work, the IRS examined new therapeutic approaches that would improve survival rates and the quality of life. The objectives of IRS-I were 1) to assess the value of postoperative radiation in children whose tumor was completely resected and who would receive vincristine, actinomycin D, and cyclophosphamide (VAC) therapy; 2) to determine the efficacy of VA compared to VAC therapy in the clinical group II patients who would each receive postoperative radiation; 3a) to assess the value of pulse-VAC therapy following local irradiation in clinical group III and IV patients; 3b) to evaluate the addition of adriamycin (Adr) to the chemotherapeutic regimen of clinical group III and IV patients.

The results of the IRS-I for GU RMS were reported in 1981 and 1982 [39,40]. Of 686 patients entered into the IRS-I, 62 patients presented with RMS arising in the bladder, prostate, or vagina. Thirty-four (55%) had all gross tumor removed at the primary operation (clinical group I). VAC therapy with or without Adr was given for 2 years in most cases. Of the 54 patients with bladder or prostate RMS, 47 (87%) were also treated with radiation therapy in doses varying from 2000 to 5500 rad. Forty-one of these 54 patients (76%) were alive and relapse free at a median of 4.5 years. Sixteen of 41 (39%) have retained their bladders. In the eight females with vaginal RMS, four were treated with radiation as well as chemotherapy. All but one patient was alive and relapse free for 4 or more years, and 6 of the 7 patients (86%) have their bladders. The overall survival rate for GU RMS reported in 1982 for IRS-I was 50 of 62 patients (81%). Relapse, either locally or with distant metastases, usually occurred within the first 2 years of treatment. Long-term survival after relapse was extremely unlikely (2 of 13 patients, 15%). The study also revealed that radiation provided no added benefit in clinical group I patients and that adriamycin did not improve the outcome of patients in clinical group III and IV.

Intergroup Rhabdomyosarcoma Study-II

The IRS-II trial of primary VAC therapy began in 1978. The objective of this study was to improve bladder salvage without altering the excellent patient survival rates previously achieved. Between 1979 and 1984, 109 patients with bladder, prostate, vaginal, uterine, and cervical tumors ("special pelvic" sites) underwent a biopsy followed by primary chemotherapy with

VAC [41]. After two chemotherapeutic cycles, the tumor response was assessed at week 8. If a tumor had diminished by 50%, two additional courses of chemotherapy were given at weeks 8 and 12. At week 16, surgical exploration was performed to determine the extent of residual disease. If there was gross or microscopic residual disease after surgical resection, radiation therapy was added to the 2 years of pulse-VAC therapy. If no residual disease was found on biopsy, the patient completed the 2-year regimen of pulse-VAC therapy. If tumor regression was less than 50% at 8 weeks, a partial cystectomy or vaginectomy was performed, providing the patient was rendered free of gross disease. If this could only be accomplished with radical cystectomy, the patient's bladder was preserved and radiation therapy was given (4000–4500 rads) for residual disease. When there was gross or microscopic residual disease after surgical resection, the patient underwent radiation therapy and continued on pulse-VAC therapy for a total of 2 years. If no residual tumor was present, the patient was maintained on pulse-VAC therapy for 2 years.

These studies showed that only about 10% of patients would be able to achieve relapse-free survival with VAC therapy alone. The majority of relapse-free survivors were patients treated with radiation when tumor regression was incomplete following chemotherapy [41]. The results of IRS-II achieved survival rates comparable to IRS-I, 70% vs. 78%, respectively. In IRS-II, only 52% of the patients had no evidence of disease at 3 years, compared to 70% of patients with disease-free status in IRS-I. Radiation therapy and/or surgery were employed to achieve these complete responses, but the primary surgical approach was the best means to achieve and maintain disease-free status. Although many patients retained their bladders initally in IRS-II as a result of the protocol design, no statistically significant difference in the percentage of patients retaining their bladder was found at 3 years between the two IRS studies (IRS-II 22% vs. IRS-I 23%). The studies demonstrated the need for improved induction chemotherapy if long-term tumor control was to be achieved. It also highlighted the importance of long-term follow-up, since 48% of patients on IRS-II were alive with preserved bladders at 1 year, whereas this percentage decreased to 33% at two years and 22% at 3 years.

Hayes et al. reported the outcome of 33/154 children with bladder RMS who underwent partial cystectomy, either as an initial procedure, a secondary procedure for localized disease following chemotherapy/irradiation, or as the initial operation when there was abdominal disease (5/33) [42]. Relapse occurred in seven of these patients (six had localized disease and an initial operation, and one had abdominal disease) who then progressed and died. The 3-year survival following partial cystectomy was similar (79%) to that for all patients with bladder RMS (78%). To date, partial cystectomy remains a surgical option but appears to be used only when gross tumor removal can be assured. Also, although the group undergoing initial partial cystectomy with known disseminated disease was small, 4/5 have remained disease free for a mean of approximately 300 weeks. This emphasizes the rationale for the use of bladder augmentation and ureteral reimplantation when indicated in the face of metastatic disease. Since most patients can have satisfactory bladder function following partial cystectomy, the recent recommendation to decrease the dose of radiation will help to prevent the development of radiation cystitis and its sequelae.

Patients on IRS-II underwent cystectomy when there was a poor response to primary chemotherapy or when local tumor progression occurred after a partial response. Also, nonresponse or progressive disease at the 8-week evaluation did not portend an unfavorable outcome with regard to survival, disease-free interval, or survival with an intact bladder when compared to patients who had complete or partial responses to chemotherapy [41].

Prognostic factors

The IRS recently reported the favorable prognostic factors in all patients with RMS [43]. The clinical group was the most important patient characteristic related to survival in both IRS-I and -II. Survival decreased from clinical group I to group IV, and in clinical group IV patients with GU tumors had significantly improved survival. Raney et al. evaluated the prognostic factors in patients with special pelvic tumors [41]. They found that children age 1–5 years had a more favorable outcome when compared with infants younger than 1 year of age. Also, patients with bladder primaries had better survival outcomes than patients with prostatic tumors. Although alveolar tumors have been recognized as having a poor prognosis when compared to embryonal, botryoid histopathology carried a significantly higher survival rate than that of the solid embryonal tumors [44]. Females had improved survival when compared to males. The 3-year survival rate for males with bladder tumors in IRS-II was 75%, while the survival rate in females was 90% (IRS-I survival 70% for females and males). Patients with prostatic tumors had a significant decrease in survival in IRS-II (59%) when compared to IRS-I (82%). The patients with prostatic tumors were somewhat older than the patients with bladder and vaginal tumors, and their tumors tended to be larger in size at the time of diagnosis. Finally, prostatic tumors were most commonly solid and not the botryoid variety. Considering all of these factors, a less favorable outcome will be predicted in this group with prostatic RMS. Therefore, primary surgery may be the best approach to ensure long-term survival in these patients [41].

Female genital tract tumors IRS-I and IRS-II

In 1988, the IRS committee reported on 47 children and adolescents with primary female genital tract tumors who were placed on IRS-I and IRS-II protocols [31]. The treatment objectives of the IRS were achieved for vaginal tumors, since pelvic exenteration is no longer performed as the initial procedure and is utilized only for complicated forms of relapse. Most of the patients were treated with initial chemotherapy followed by delayed hysterectomy and/or partial vaginectomy. Hysterectomy continues to be the standard approach in more than 50% of patients with tumors originating in the proximal portion of the vagina. At least one ovary is retained in most patients and repositioned to avoid irradiation effects. Six relapses occured in 26 patients with localized vaginal tumors. Five patients who relapsed were free of disease for a mean of 4.4 years following salvage chemotherapy. The 19 patients without disease recurrence have been followed for a mean of 5.4 years.

Ten patients who presented with uterine sarcomas underwent chemotherapy [31]. Those with localized polypoid lesions had disease amenable to polypectomy with or without dilation and currettage. These patients have remained disease free (2.5–6.5 years), while four patients with more extensive uterine infiltration or penetration into the abdominal cavity and/or metastatic disease died within the first year after the initiation of therapy. Also, it has been difficult, especially in the infant group, to determine the precise site of the primary tumor in patients where the origin appears to be the vagina or uterus. In this group of patients, primary uterine tumors occurred almost exclusively in the adolescent or postadolescent females, thereby making the vaginal origin in the infant or prepubertal female more common.

Vulvar tumors have been managed with resection and chemotherapy with or without adjunctive radiation therapy [31]. Eight of nine patients were disease free, with a mean of 6.4 years, while one patient had recurrent disease at 2.5 years.

Intergroup Rhabdomyosarcoma Study-III

The objectives of the IRS-III study were to answer the following questions: 1) Can chemotherapy be reduced to only 1 year of VA therapy in patients with clinical group I and II "favorable" histology? 2) What is the role of additional cisplatin and adriamycin in pulse-VAC therapy? 3) Will the addition of cisplatin or cisplatin plus etoposide (VP-16) to VAC improve the complete response and relapse-free survival interval in patients in clinical groups III-IV? 4) Will second- and third-look surgery to pathologically confirm the efficacy of therapy improve the ultimate local control in patients in clinical groups III and IV? 5) In patients achieving only a partial response by week 20, will more intense chemotherapy with adriamycin, dicarbazine (DTIC), or dactinomycin and VP-16 or dactinomycin plus DTIC improve the survival outcome [45]?

To date, the IRS-III protocol results utilizing repetitive pulse-VAC therapy as the control, and repetitive pulse-VAdrC-VAC *plus* cisplatin vs. repetitive pulse-VAdrC-VAC *plus* cisplatin *plus* VP-16 are preliminary [46].

Although survival and the complete response duration have increased significantly throughout the years of the three IRS protocols (overall updated survival rates were 73% in IRS-III, 67% in IRS-II, and 60% in IRS-I, and complete response rates were 76% vs. 69% vs. 64%, respectively), it does not appear to be due to the superiority of either experimental regimen over the control therapy. The data involving patients with only genitourinary tumors on IRS-III have not been published.

Intergroup Rhabdomyosarcoma Study-IV

Based upon the observations from IRS-I and IRS-III, new objectives have been proposed for IRS-IV [47]. The goals of IRS-IV are to compare the survival rates of patients receiving VAC vs. vincristine-actinomycin D-ifosfamide (VAI) vs. vincristine-ifosfamide-etoposide (VIE). Also hyperfractionated radiation therapy (Hyperfx-RT) will be compared to conventional therapy. Conventional radiation is delivered as 180 rads in 28 fractions for a total of 5040 rads over $5\frac{1}{2}$ weeks. Hyperfractionated radiation is given twice a day at 6- to 8-hour intervals for a total of 5940s rads in 54 fractions of 110 rads each. This is being investigated to evaluate the local control rate in clinical group III patients only, since group II patients have previously had an acceptable local control rate with conventional therapy.

In patients on the IRS-IV protocols with genitourinary tumors, bladder salvage can be anticipated in 25–45% of patients based on the IRS-II data and preliminary data from IRS-III [47]. As long as a partial response is seen, radical extirpative surgery should be delayed. The patient follows the designated therapy of the appropriate protocol. If there is biopsy-proven residual tumor at 6 months after completing radiation therapy or progressive disease is noted after the initiating of chemotherapy and radiation therapy, a partial cystectomy, when possible, is performed or an anterior exenteration is indicated. Survival is not adversely affected if radical surgery is delayed until residual tumor is defined or progression is noted, but further delay is not recommended. In patients undergoing partial cystectomy, ureteral reimplantation may be indicated. Bladder augmentation has been employed even in patients with metastatic disease. The role of continent urinary diversion has not been defined in a large series of patients to date. In patients requiring only radical prostatectomy, the ability to preserve the urethra and bladder is unusual when there has been a poor response to chemotherapy. In males undergoing radical prostatectomy or radical cystoprostatectomy, a urologic surgeon who is skilled in preserving the neurovascular bundles for potency should participate in the surgery if this would not leave gross residual tumor [48].

The IRS-IV also addresses the approach to female genital tract tumors [47]. Some polypoid tumors of the uterus can be excised without hysterectomy. When hysterectomy is performed for a uterine tumor, preservation of the distal vagina and ovaries is generally indicated. When the tumor occurs in the distal vagina, hysterectomy is not required. Proximal vaginal tumors may necessitate hysterectomy with partial or complete vaginectomy. Anterior exenteration is usually not necessary for tumor removal, but when indicated is an effective means of local control.

In clinical group IV patients with female genital tract tumors, primary chemotherapy and/or radiation therapy is administered and no interval radical surgery is performed [47]. When patients are free of metastatic disease for 3–6 months, surgical intervention should occur if there is biopsy-proven residual disease or progression of local disease occurs with the initiation of chemo and radiation therapy.

The drugs used on the IRS-IV protocol have been associated with adverse hematologic effects, usually reversible myelosuppression. In addition, ifosfamide and cyclophosphamide should be withheld when there is significant microscopic hematuria (greater than 50 RBC/HPF). When the hematuria resolves, the doses are decreased to 50% for 1 week and then increased to the normal level. MESNA therapy, which binds the acrolein metabolite of those agents that led to severe hemorrhagic cystitis and late-occurring bladder carcinomas in the past, is utilized. In addition, the chemotherapy can also cause severe peripheral neuritis or paralytic ileus. The neurologic abnormalities, including seizures, are most commonly seen with ifosfamide and vincristine. Since RMS is generally a disease of early childhood, it is too early to know the long-term deleterious effects of therapy in this group of patients. It is important to perform surveillance in this group to assure that their growth and development, including gonadal function, is normal [49,50]. Long-term follow-up is imperative in view of the risk of a second malignancy following treatment for other childhood cancers [51].

Paratesticular rhabdomyosarcoma

Paratesticular RMS comprises approximately 7% of all RMS [1]. These tumors arise from the distal spermatic cord and may invade the testis or surrounding tunics. The most common histopathology of these tumors is embryonal (97%) [52].

The initial operative procedure is a radical orchiectomy. This is performed through an inguinal incision with initial proximal vascular control. If a biopsy is indicated, the area should be draped off from the operative field to avoid spillage and contamination. Transcrotal procedures should be avoided to prevent the likelihood of contamination. A metastatic evaluation is performed that includes a CT of the chest and abdomen, since lymphatic spread is seen in approximately 28% [52]. A bone scan or skeletal survey is recommended, as well as a bone-marrow aspirate and/or biopsy. The IRS surgical pathologic staging and treatment is defined in Table 2 [53].

There continues to be controversy regarding the need for retroperitoneal lymph-node dissection (RPLND) following the diagnosis of paratesticular RMS and before the initiation of chemotherapy. Nodal involvement was

Table 2. IRS-IV staging and treatment of paratesticular rhabdomyosarcoma

Clinical Group	Tumor Status	Therapy
I	Tumor completely excised[a] (not alveolar subtype)	Vincristine Actinomycin D (VA) for 1 year[b]
II	Tumor excised with microscopic residual disease at margin and/or positive lymph nodes involving the ipsilateral hilar-paraaortic chain	VAC vs. VAI for 1–2 years plus radiation[c] therapy to involved region
III	Gross residual local and/or regional disease (retroperitoneal nodes) that is not surgical removable	3–7 drug regimen plus radiation[d] therapy to involved region
IV	Distant metastases	Same as Group III

[a] If there has been scrotal contamination, hemiscrotectomy and relocation of the testis into the thigh is advised to avoid the effects of local radiation on the remaining gonad.
[b] No radiation for Group I patients.
[c] Conventional radiation.
[d] Conventional or hyperfractionated radiation.

found in 28% of 77 cases of localized paratesticular sarcoma from IRS-I and IRS-II. Since only radiation is given to clinical group II, the pathologic status of these nodes is important. With the additional radiation therapy, clinical group II patients have a 90% relapse-free survival for at least 2 years [52].

Olive et al. reporting on the European experience with the International Society of Pediatic Oncology (SIOP) protocol, suggest that RLND is not needed if the clinical examination, CT, and ultrasound, or bipedal lymph-angiography do not demonstrate retroperitoneal disease [54]. Chemotherapy alone, consisting of VIA, has more recently been used [55]. The current recommendation of the IRS is to perform an ipsilateral RLN sampling, which will preserve the lumbar sympathetic nerves involved in ejaculation, therefore preserving potential fertility [53,56].

Further attempts at ensuring potential fertility include the avoidance of alkylating agents (cylophosphamide) in clinical group I patients, since these agents have known adverse effects on sperm production. Since the cure rate is 93% in group I and 90% in Group II, fertility potential is an important concern of these patients and their families [52].

Results of therapy

Overall survival in the 95 patients entered into IRS-I and IRS-II with paratesticular RMS was 89% at 3 years. Most of the patients were in clinical group I (60%) and II (21%). Only one patient from group I and two patients from group II developed recurrent sarcoma. In groups III and IV, 7/18 developed progressive disease, but despite this, 11/18 are alive at 3 years. Early results from IRS-III do not show any significant differences in relapse rates to date [52].

Although much progress has been made in the therapy of RMS, with survival rates of 65–89% reported, an 11–35% mortality still exists. La Quaglia et al. performed a retropective analysis of 28 males with paratesticular embryonal RMS, examining factors that may have predicted a fatal outcome [57]. Univariate analysis revealed two significant factors: 1) resectability, that is, the presence of unresectable retroperitoneal disease in the absence of distant metastases and 2) the presence of distant metastases at the time of diagnosis. Unresectability appeared to be the most important predictor of mortality and may suggest that these patients represent a subset requiring more aggressive therapy, such as myeloablative regimens with bone marrow transplantation.

The multimodal management of children with RMS of the GU tract continues to present challenges to all who are involved in the care of these young patients. We are grateful for the dedication of the IRS committee members and participating institutions who continue to devote their efforts toward improving the lives of children with RMS.

References

1. Young JL, Miller RW: Incidence of malignant tumors in United States children. J Pediatr 86:254, 1975.
2. Stout AP: Rhabdomyosarcoma of the skeletal muscles. Ann Surg 123:447, 1946.
3. Thompson IM, Coppridge AJ: The management of bladder tumors in children: A study of sarcoma botryoides. J Urol 82:390–395, 1959.
4. Higgins TT: Rhabdomyosarcoma of the bladder. Br J Urol 24:158, 1952.
5. Kramer SA, Kelalis PP: Pediatric urologic oncology. In: Gillenwater JY, Grayhack JT, Howards SS, Duckett JW (eds). *Adult and Pediatric Urology*, 2nd ed. Mosby-Year Book, St. Louis, 1987, pp. 2268–2273.
6. Maurer HM, Moen T, Donaldson M et al.: The Intergroup Rhabdomyosarcoma Study: A preliminary report. Cancer 40:2015–2026, 1977.
7. Pizzo PA, Horowitz ME, Peplack DG, Hays DM, Kun LE: Solid tumors of childhood. In: DeVita VT Jr., Hellman S, Rosenberg SA (eds). *Cancer: Principles and Practice of Oncology*. Philadelphia, J.B. Lippincott, 1989, pp. 1647–1654.
8. Li FP, Fraumeni JR Jr.: Soft tissue sarcomas, breast cancer and other neoplasms: A family cancer syndrome. Ann Intern Med 71:747–752, 1969.
9. Douglass EC, Valentine M, Etcubanas E, Parham D, Webber BL, Houghton DJ, Houghton JA, Green AA: A specific chromosomal abnormality in rhabdomyosarcoma. Cytogenet Cell Genet 45:148–155, 1987.
10. Intergroup Rhabdomyosarcoma Study laboratory evaluation of tumor tissue, Nov 1990, pp. 1–8.
11. Houghton JA, Meyer WH, Houghton PJ: Scheduling of vincristine: Drug accumulation and response of demographics of childhood rhabdomyosarcoma determined by frequency of administration. Cancer Treat Rep 71:717–721, 1987.

12. Roberts WM, Douglass EC, Peiper SC, Look AT: Amplification of the GLI gene in childhood sarcomas. Cancer Res 49:5407–5413, 1989.
13. Schwab M, Alitalo K, Klempnauer K-H, Varmus HE, Bishop JM, Gilbert F, Brodeur G, Goldstein M, Trent J: Amplified DNA with limited homology to MYC cellular oncogene is shared by human neuroblastoma cell lines and a neuroblastoma tumor. Nature (London) 305:245–248, 1983.
14. Mitani K, Kurosawa H, Suzuki A, Hayashi Y, Hanada R, Tamaoto K, Domatsu A, Kobayashi N, Nakagome Y, Yamada M: Amplification of N-myc in a rhabdomyosarcoma. Jpn J Cancer Res 77:1062–1065, 1986.
15. Garson JA, Clayton J, McIntyre PG, Kemshead JT: N-myc oncogene amplification in rhabdomyosarcoma at relapse. Lancet 2:1496, 1986.
16. Boyle ET Jr., Reiman HM, Kramer SA, Kelalis PP, Rainwater LM, Lieber MM: Embryonal rhabdomyosarcoma of bladder and prostate: Nuclear DNA pattern studied by flow cytometry. J Urol 14:1119–1121, 1988.
17. Mostofi FK, Morse WM: Polypoid rhabdomyosarcoma (sarcoma botryoides) of bladder in children. J Urol 67:681–687, 1952.
18. Batsakis JG: Urogenital rhabdomyosarcoma: Histogenesis and classification. J Urol 90:180, 1963.
19. Stout AP, Lattes R: Tumors of the soft tissues. In: *Atlas of Tumor Pathology*, Fascicle 1, Second Series. Armed Forces Institute of Pathology, Washington, DC, 1967, pp. 134–144.
20. Lawrence W, Hayes DM: Surgical lesions from the Intergroup Rhabdomyosarcoma Study. Natl Cancer Inst Monogr 56:159–162, 1981.
21. Grosfeld JL, Weber TR, Weetman RM, Bachner RL: Rhabdomyosarcoma in childhood: Analysis of survival in 98 cases. J Pediatr Surg 18(2):141–146, 1983.
22. Tefft J, Jaffe N: Sarcoma of the bladder and prostate in children. Cancer 32:1161–1171, 1973.
23. Gaiger AM, Soule EH, Newton WA Jr.: Pathology of rhabdomyosarcoma: Experience of the Intergroup Rhabdomyosarcoma Study, Natl Cancer Inst Monogr 56:19, 1981.
24. Horn RC, Enterline HT: Rhabdomyosarcoma: A clinicopathologic study and classification in 39 cases. Cancer 11:181–191, 1958.
25. Patton RB, Horn RC Jr.: Rhabdomyosarcoma: Clinical and pathological features and comparisons with human fetal and embryonal skeletal muscle. Surgery 52:572, 1962.
26. Mahour GH, Soule EH, Mills SD, Lynn HB: Rhabdomyosarcoma in infants and children: A clinicopathologic study of 75 cases. J Pediatr Surg 2:402, 1967.
27. Children's Cancer Study Group: Protocol CCG-212: Intergroup Rhabdomyosarcoma Study-III.
28. Hayes DM, Raney RB Jr., Lawrence W Jr., Tefft M, Soule EH, Crist WM, Foulkes M, Maurer H: Primary chemotherapy in the treatment of children with bladder-prostate tumors in the Intergroup Rhabdomyosarcoma Study (IRS-II). J Pediatr Surg 17:812, 1982.
29. Snyder HM, D'Anglio GJ, Evans AE, Raney RB: Pediatric urology In: Walsh PC, Gittes RF, Perlmutter AD, Stamey TA (eds). *Campbell's Urology*, 5th ed, WB Saunders, Philadelphia, 1986, chap 57.
30. Lawrence W Jr., Hayes DM, Heyn R, Tefft M, Crist W, Beltangady M, Newton W Jr., Wharam M: Lymphatic metastases with childhood rhabdomyosarcoma. Cancer 60:910–915, 1987.
31. Hays DM, Shimada H, Raney RB, Tefft M, Newton W, Crist W, Lawrence W Jr., Ragab A, Beltangady M, Maurer H: Clinical staging and treatment results in rhabdomyosarcoma of the female genital tract among children and adolescence. Cancer 61:1893–1903, 1988.
32. Sty JR, Wells RG: Other abdominal and pelvic masses in children. Semin Roentgenol 23:216–231, 1988.
33. Hahn: Neoplasms of the urinary bladder. In: Pollack H (ed). *Clinical Urography*, Vol 2, W.B. Saunders, Philadelphia, 1990, chap 46.
34. Maurer HM, Moon T, Donaldson M, Fernandez C, Gehan EA, Hammond D, Hays DM: The Intergroup Rhabdomyosarcoma Study: A preliminary report. Cancer 40:2015, 1977.

35. Green DM, Jaffe N: Progress and controversy in the treatment of childhood rhabdomyosarcoma. Cancer Treat Rev 5:7, 1978.
36. Stobbe GC, Dargeon HW: Embryonal rhabdomyosarcoma of the head and neck in children and adolescents. Cancer 3:826, 1950.
37. D'Angio GJ, Farber S, Maddock CL: Potentiation of x-ray effect by actinomycin D. Radiology 73:175, 1959.
38. Pinkel D, Pickren J: Rhabdomyosarcoma in children. JAMA 175:293, 1961.
39. Hays DM, Raney RB Jr., Lawrence W Jr., Gehan EA, Soule EH, Tefft M, Maurer HM: Rhabdomyosarcoma of the female urogenital tract. J Pediatr Surg 16:828–834, 1981.
40. Hays DM, Raney RB Jr., Lawrence W Jr., Soule EH, Gehan EA, Tefft M: Bladder and prostatic tumors in the Intergroup Rhabdomyosarcoma Study: Results of therapy. Cancer 50:1472–1482, 1982.
41. Raney RB Jr., Gehan EA, Hays DM, Tefft M, Newton W Jr., Haeberlen V, Maurer H: Primary chemotherapy with or without radiation therapy and/or surgery for children with localized sarcoma of the bladder, prostate, vagina, uterus and cervix. Cancer 66:2072–2081, 1990.
42. Hayes DM, Lawrence W Jr., Crist W, Weiner CE, Raney RB Jr., Ragab A, Tefft M, Webber B, Johnston J, Maurer H: Partial cystectomy in the management of rhabdomyosarcoma of the bladder: A report from the Intergroup Rhabdomyosarcoma Study. J Pediatr Surg 25:719–723, 1990.
43. Crist WM, Garnsey L, Beltangady MS, Gehan E, Ruymann F, Webber B, Hays D, Wharam M, Maurer H: Prognosis in children with rhabdomyosarcoma: A report of the Intergroup Rhabdomyosarcoma Studies I and II. J Clin Oncol 8:443–452, 1990.
44. Ghazali S: Embryonic rhabdomyosarcoma in the urogenital tract. Br J Surg 60:124, 1973.
45. Intergoup Rhabdomyosarcoma Study III, November 1984.
46. Maurer H, Gehan E, Crist W, Morris-Jones P, Newton W, Ortega J, Wiener E, Wharam M: Intergroup Rhabdomyosarcoma Study III: A preliminary report of overall outcome. Proc Am Soc Clinc Oncol 8:296, 1989.
47. Intergroup Rhabdomyosarcoma Study IV for stage 2 and 3 disease, November 1990.
48. Brendler CB, Steinberg GD, Marshall FF, Mostwin JL, Walsh PC: Local recurrence and survival following nerve-sparing radical cystoprostectomy. J Urol 144:1137, 1990.
49. Silber JH, Litman PS, Meadows AT: Stature loss folllowing skeletal irradiation for childhood cancer. J Clin Oncol 8:304, 1990.
50. Aubier F, Flamant F, Brauner R, Caillaud JM, Chaussain JM, Lemerle J: Male gonadal function after chemotherapy for solid tumors in childhood. J Clin Oncol 7:304, 1989.
51. Meadows AT, Obringer AC, Marrero O, Oberlin O, Robison L, Fossati-Bellani F, Green D, Voute PA: Second malignant neoplasms following childhood Hodgkins's disease treatment and splenectomy as risk factors. Med Pediatr Oncol 17(6):477, 1989.
52. Raney RB Jr., Tefft M, Lawrence W Jr., Ragab AH, Soule EH, Beltangady M, Gehan EA: Paratesticular sarcoma in childhood and adolescence: A report from the Intergroup Rhabdomyosarcoma Studies I and II, 1973–1983. Cancer 60:2337–2343, 1987.
53. Intergroup Rhabdomyosarcoma Study IV for stage I disease, November 1990.
54. Olive D, Flamant F, Zucker JM, Voute P, Brunat-Mentigny M, Otten J, Dutou L: Paraaortic lymphadenectomy is not necessary in the treatment of localized paratesticular rhabdomyosarcoma. Cancer 54:1283–1287, 1984.
55. Olive-Sommelet D: International Society of Pediatric Oncology protocol. Dialog Ped Urol 12:4–5, 1989.
56. Rowland R, Donohue J: Scrotum and testis. In: Gillenwater JY, Grayhack JT, Howards SS, Duckett JW (eds). *Adult and Pediatric Urology*, 2nd ed. Mosby-Year Book, St. Louis, 1987, pp. 1576–1590.
57. LaQuaglia MP, Fereshteh H, Heller G, Herr H, Mandell LR, Corbally M, Hajdu S, Exelby P: Mortality in pediatric paratesticular rhabdomyosarcoma: A multivariate analysis. J Urol 142:473–478, 1989.

2. Renal-sparing surgery for renal and transitional cell carcinoma

Russell K. Lawson

Renal-sparing surgery for kidney tumors has received considerable attention over the past several years, with some authors suggesting that such procedures may be carried out in patients with a normal contralateral kidney [1]. There are obvious indications for renal-sparing procedures in patients with a solitary kidney or bilateral renal tumors, but with a few minor exceptions such a treatment plan has not been proven safe in patients with a normal opposite kidney. In this chapter I will present the counterevidence to this ultraistic point of view, as well as a discussion of the procedures currently used to to manage bilateral tumors or tumors in a solitary kidney.

Renal cell carcinoma

Renal cell carcinoma is the commonest indication for renal-sparing surgery in patients with a solitary kidney or bilateral tumors. The tumor-free survival is fair to good following these procedures, depending on the number, size, location, grade, and stage of the tumors [2–6]. Because of reasonable outcomes following these procedures, it is tempting to speculate that partial nephrectomy or enucleation of the tumor in patients with small renal-cell carcinomas would be a good alternative to radical nephrectomy. Three papers have been published that strongly mitigate against renal-sparing surgery unless absolutely necessary. The first is a paper by Mukamel and coworkers, who carefully examined 66 kidneys that had been removed for clinically evident renal-cell carcinoma to determine the incidence of occult tumors [7]. They found 58 tumors in 20 kidneys, ranging in size from 1 to 15 mm. These authors used histologic criteria, previously published by Mostafi, to distinguish between benign adenomas and renal cell carcinomas. Using these criteria, they found that seven kidneys contained benign adenomas, nine kidneys contained renal cell carcinomas, and four contained both benign and malignant nodules. From the original group of 66 kidneys removed for overt carcinoma, 13 or 20% contained occult nodules of renal cell carcinoma. Five of the occult carcinomas had a histologic pattern identical with the primary tumor. The authors were not able to determine

Lepor, H. and Lawson R.K., (eds.), Therapy for Genitourinary Cancer. *ISBN 0-7923-1412-3.*

whether these lesions were de novo tumors that occurred in other areas of the kidney, similar to the field effect seen in some bladder cancers, or whether they represented metastases from the primary tumor. This study also does not provide information on the incidence of occult tumors in the contralateral kidney. Nevertheless, the high incidence of occult tumors in the ipisilateral kidney indicates that approximately one fifth of the patients who undergo a renal-sparing procedure are likely to have tumor remaining in the kidney.

The other two papers bearing on this topic were published by Marshall and coworkers and Blackley et al., regarding the effectiveness of tumor enucleation in eliminating all renal cell carcinoma from the kidney [8, 9]. The results of these two studies are similar. Blackley carried out a nephrectomy in 25 patients and a partial nephrectomy in one patient for renal cell carcinoma. The surgical specimens were then subjected to extracorporeal resection of the primary tumor. Histopathological examination of the kidney following a careful attempt to remove all tumor by enucleation revealed that 42% of the kidneys had retained tumor. Failure to remove all tumor was due to the following factors: Residual tumor in the bed of the enucleation (7), microscopic capsular or venous invasion (3), tumor thrombus extending into retained vein (1), and multifocal tumors (3).

Two recent series of patients treated conservatively for renal cell carcinoma have appeared in the literature. Novick and coworkers described a series of 100 patients who had renal-sparing surgery, and only four patients in this series had normal contralateral kidneys [6]. The authors cautioned that renal-sparing surgery in this setting has not been proven safe and that radical nephrectomy is the treatment of choice. The second paper by Morgan and Zincke describes the outcome of renal-sparing surgery in 104 patients. [10]. Twenty patients in this series had normal contralateral kidneys. The authors state that all 20 of the patients had small, low-stage and low-grade tumors. However, it has been previously shown that not all small tumors are low grade [11]. Furthermore, stage and grade can only be determined accurately from histopathological examination of the surgical specimen. This retrospective information is of little value in selecting the appropriate surgical procedure in a given case. These authors report a mean follow-up of 3.85 years in this subgroup of 20 patients, which is too short a time to provide meaningful data regarding the efficacy of renal-sparing surgery in patients with a normal contralateral kidney. One of the conclusions from this paper states that renal-sparing surgery in patients with a normal contralateral kidney is not recommended for general use and should be considered investigational.

The problems with the series of patients reported to date are the following: 1) Too few patients with normal contralateral kidneys treated with renal-sparing procedures; 2) too short a follow-up to determine the efficacy of the procedure; and 3) lack of information regarding the natural history of this disease. This last shortcoming is of major importance. There is no doubt that renal-sparing surgery is safe and effective in some patients with a normal contralateral kidney.

The paper referred to earlier by Mukamel demonstrated a high incidence of occult tumors in kidneys removed for clinically apparent renal cell carcinoma. Theoretically, this finding means that a high number of patients treated for renal cell carcinoma with renal-sparing procedures will develop recurrence in the ipisilateral kidney. However, the recurrence rate is considerably lower than predicted. This discrepancy is most likely due to the variability in the growth rate of these tumor and/or a lack of understanding of why some renal cell carcinomas remain dormant and why some grow rapidly [12–14]. Until there is a better understanding of the natural history of this disease, radical nephrectomy remains the treatment of choice in patients with a normal opposite kidney.

An opposite treatment plan is best for patients with Von Hippl Lindau disease, where the incidence of multiple asynchronous tumors in both kidneys is high [15–17]. Renal cell carcinomas in patients with this disease tend to be low grade. Consequently, as much renal tissue as possible should be spared, which generally can be achieved by enucleation of the tumor.

Patients who have a solitary kidney, bilateral tumors, or a poorly functioning kidney with a contralateral renal tumor should be managed, if possible, by renal-sparing surgery. The surgical options include bilateral nephrectomy, unilateral nephrectomy with a contralateral renal-sparing procedure, bilateral renal-sparing procedures, or a renal-sparing procedure in patients with a solitary kidney. The renal-sparing procedures are a partial nephrectomy, tumor enucleation, and extracorporeal surgery.

The first report of extracorporeal renal surgery for renal cell carcinoma was by Calne in 1971 [18]. A patient with a large renal-cell carcinoma in a solitary kidney underwent extracorporeal resection of the tumor followed by autotransplantation. In 1971, Gelin and associates described two patients treated for renal cell carcinoma by extracorporeal resection of the tumor and autotransplantation [19]. Following these early reports, a number of papers appeared describing the use of this technique for managing renal cell carcinoma in a solitary kidney [20–23]. The initial enthusiasm for this surgical approach was tempered by a high incidence of serious renal damage or renal failure associated with the procedure [6]. At the present time, there is a limited place for extracorporeal surgery and autotransplantation to treat renal cell carcinoma in a solitary kidney.

When the tumor is large and central in the kidney, and particularly if resection of the tumor requires extensive vascular reconstruction, then extracorporeal surgery may be the best procedure for the patient. The advantages of extracorporeal surgery over in situ resection of the tumor are the safe extension of ischemic operating time by cold preservation, the use of high magnification to carry out vessel repair, complete renal mobility for improved vessel and collecting system repair, and decreased blood loss. The major disadvantages are an increased risk of renal injury, particularly in older patients with some degree of nephrosclerosis, and the added risk of complications from the additional procedure of autotransplantation.

An appropriately selected case of extracorporeal surgery for a large central renal cell carcinoma is illustrated in Figure 1. This patient presented with gross hematuria and was found to have a large renal cell carcinoma in a solitary kidney. Nephrectomy was carried out, and the kidney was perfused and cooled with chilled preservation solution. Extracorporeal excision of the tumor was carried with the kidney maintained at 7° Centigrade in an ice bath. Multiple biopsies were taken from the resected tumor bed and examined by frozen section. A tongue of tumor measuring 3 × 5 mm was discovered and resected. The kidney was then autotransplanted into the right groin. The patient is currently free of tumor $8\frac{1}{2}$ years following surgery, with a serum creatinine of 3.0 mg/dl.

When a renal cell carcinoma is enucleated, whether in situ or as an extracorporeal procedure, an attempt should be made to remove a rim of

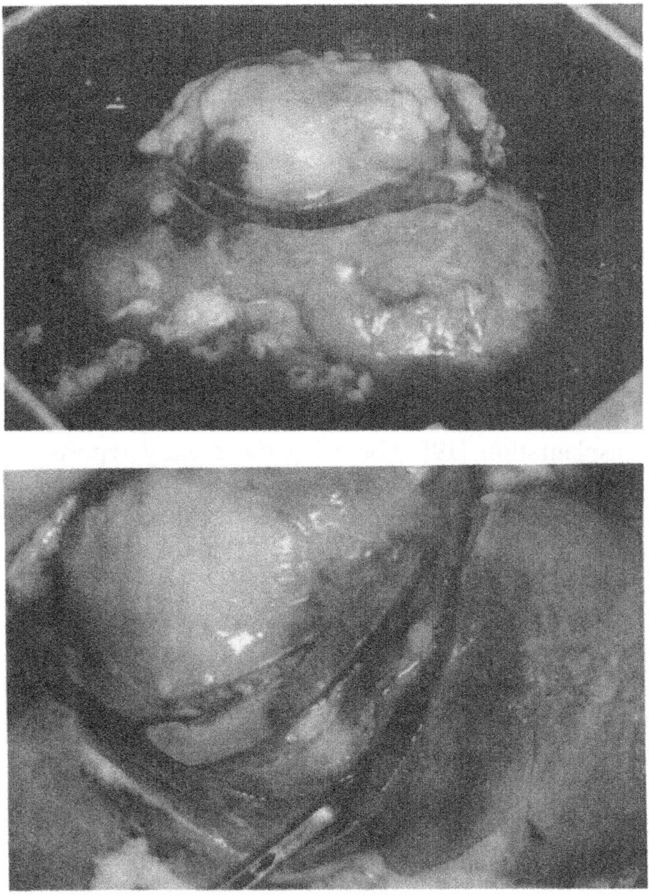

A

B

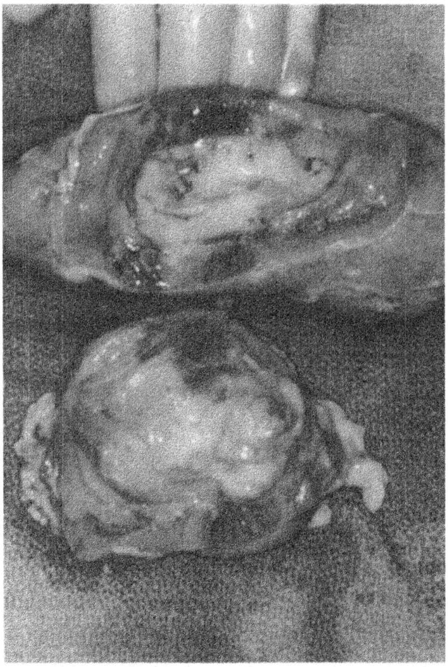

C

Figure 1. Extracorporeal surgery for renal cell carcinoma in a solitary kidney. A: Kidney in ice bath. The line of incision between the tumor mass and the kidney is shown. B: Separation of tumor from normal renal tissue. The tumor pseudocapsule can be seen. C: Tumor completely resected and remaining normal kidney.

normal tissue along with the pseudocapsule. The work by Blackley and coworkers has shown that the pseudocapsule surrounding a tumor may vary in thickness and that in about one fourth of the cases tumor will be left behind, even when an attempt is made to remove a substantial margin of surrounding normal kidney tissue [9]. Careful inspection of the tumor bed under moderate magnification with biopsy and frozen section of any suspicious areas is required. Some authors advocate frozen-section examination of the surface of the resected tumor to assist in locating breaches of the pseudocapsule.

The enucleation procedure can be carried out with a flexible, blunt probe. When small-and medium-size arteries are encountered, they resist tearing with the probe and can often be identified, ligated, and transected as the dissection progresses. I have found that microvessel clips work well for this purpose, as long as care is taken not to place them immediately adjacent to an opening in the collecting system where they might become a nidus for stone formation. Openings in the collecting system and venous system can be located by gently perfusing the renal vein and ureter under low pressure with chilled perfusate. If the procedure is being carried out in situ, both the vein and ureter can be cannulated with a small needle to deliver the perfusate. The veins and open arteries should be closed with 7–0 non-absorbable vascular suture and the collecting system with fine absorbable suture material.

Operating time can be substantially increased with a decreased risk of ischemic renal injury during in situ procedures by cooling the kidney with saline slush after isolation and clamping of the renal artery and vein. I prefer to heparinize the patient several minutes before clamping the renal vessels. The effect of systemic heparin on wound bleeding is usually not a problem, but if troublesome oozing occurs, the systemic heparinization can be reversed with protamine after clamping the renal artery. Those patients who remain systemically heparinized during the procedure are reversed with protamine prior to closure of the incision. Occasionally, there is a substantial retrograde arterial flow through the ureteral artery that necessitates the placement of a soft clamp across the ureter during the procedure. Following enucleation of the tumor, the remaining renal parenchyma can be folded into apposition, and the capsule covering the upper and lower poles can be sutured together to provide better hemostasis.

Whenever possible, a partial nephrectomy should be carried out, instead of tumor enucleation. Partial nephrectomy is particularly applicable for polar lesions. An arteriogram is helpful in planning the renal incision to ensure the best possible arterial blood supply to the remaining normal segment of kidney tissue. Microvascular repair, including interposition of autologous arterial grafts, may be necessary to preserve good blood supply. A margin of at least 1 cm of normal parenchyma should be removed with the specimen to reduce the risk of tumor infiltration of the surgical margin. The larger open arteries and veins on the surface of the kidney should be ligated, clipped, or sutured. The Beacon Laboratories Argon Coagulator is helpful for controlling any residual bleeding on the cut surface of the kidney. Frozen section of the margin of the specimen should be carried out to ensure adequate tumor resection.

Partial nephrectomy can either be carried out with in situ cooling following clamping of the renal vessels or without interrupting renal circulation. If the latter course is selected, then tapes should be placed around the renal artery and vein to ensure vascular control if excessive bleeding occurs. Partial nephrectomy without clamping the renal vessels is least likely to result in ischemic injury to the remaining normal renal tissue but does substantially increase blood loss over the alternative method. The raw surface of the kidney may be covered with Gelfoam, Surgicel, or perinephric fat, which is held in place by suturing the material to the remaining renal capsule.

Transitional cell carcinoma

Transitional cell carcinoma of the kidney is less common than renal cell carcinoma and accounts for only 6–7% of all renal tumors. However, because of a relatively high incidence of recurrent tumors on the ipsilateral side in patients treated by renal-sparing surgery and poor tumor-free survival in patients with high-grade tumors, the surgical management of this problem is controversial. In 1933, Kimball and Ferris reviewed the problem of ipsilateral ureteral recurrence following nephrectomy for transitional cell carcinoma of the renal pelvis and recommended nephroureterectomy with excision of a cuff of bladder for this disease. [24]. Since that time, nephroureterectomy with a cuff of bladder has become the standard procedure for transitional cell carcinoma of the upper urinary tract. Renal-sparing surgery for this tumor is generally accepted only if there is contralateral renal disease, synchronous bilateral tumors, or a solitary kidney. Several papers have appeared in recent years advocating a more thoughtful approach to this problem [25–27]. A number of factors have resulted in a reassessment of the need to remove the kidney in all patients with transitional cell carcinoma of the renal pelvis who have a normal contralateral kidney. The most important of these factors is diagnostic retrograde ureteroscopy. Small flexible, steerable ureteroscopes are now available that allow inspection of the entire upper urinary tract in over 90% of patients. [26,28]. Biopsy of suspicious areas of mucosa can be accomplished with these instruments. The addition of CT scanning and urine cytology to the IVP and retrograde pyelogram in the workup of these patients has also reduced the risk of missing a high-grade infiltrating tumor of the renal pelvis. Some authors are now advocating renal-sparing procedures in patients who have low-grade, low-stage, upper urinary tract transitional cell carcinoma and a normal opposite kidney [25–27,29]. Lesions that appear to be high grade or infiltrating by ureteropyeloscopy in patients who do not have a normal contralateral kidney should be treated by renal-sparing surgery only if it appears that the tumor can be completely resected. High-grade invasive tumors in patients with renal disease or a solitary kidney are best treated by nephroureterectomy and chronic dialysis. Although there is relatively little information regarding the efficacy of M-VAC in the management of stage 2–4 transitional cell carcinoma of the renal pelvis, it seems likely that tumor response rates should correspond closely with those attained with bladder tumors [30]. Adjuvent chemotherapy may well influence the treatment plan for these tumors in the future.

The two major reasons why renal-sparing surgery for transitional cell carcinoma of the renal pelvis is not generally accepted are the high incidence of ipsilateral recurrence and the concern that opening the collecting system will seed tumor cells into the perinephric space [26,27,31,32]. Preoperative ureteropyeloscopy with a small, flexible ureteroscope greatly reduces the risk of inadvertently opening the collecting system in the presence of high-grade tumor. The second concern of local seeding of tumor cells remains problematic. In the case of bladder tumors, partial cystectomy does not appear to result in a high incidence of wound seeding [33]. If this same phenomenon applies to upper tract tumors, then the risk of local spread appears to be low if endoscopically low-grade tumors are treated by percutaneous nephroscopy and electroresection and/or laser fulgeration. Laser fulgeration through a flexible ureteroscope has also been used to successfully treat low-grade ureteral and renal pelvis tumors [27,34].

These procedures have not been established as efficacious and the risk of tumor seeding from percutaneous procedures is not known. There is also the theoretical risk of local tumor spread from pyelointersitial backflow if intraoperative pelvic pressure exceeds 10–15 cm of water during endoscopy. At the present time, the most accepted procedure for management of these tumors in patients without a normal contralateral kidney is partial nephrectomy. If the lesion is located in a calyx, the infudibulum to the calyx can be isolated and ligated, followed by a partial nephrectomy of that segment [25]. Pyeloscopy with a rigid or flexible instrument can then be carried out to ensure that the remainder of the collecting system is free of tumor. Lesions of the renal pelvis are more of a problem, because resection of more than a small piece of pelvic wall leaves a defect that must be covered. I have found that modest-sized defects can be covered with a piece of renal capsule. Large defects can be closed by interposition of an isolated ileal segment. Surgical margins should be checked by frozen section before closing the collecting system. Careful packing and isolation of the renal pelvis from the perinephric space with lap sponges is thought to minimize the risk of seeding of the wound during resection of the tumor.

Renal-sparing procedures for transitional cell carcinoma of the renal pelvis are gaining favor in carefully selected cases because of improved ability to clinically grade and stage the lesion by ureteropyeloscopy. Small low-grade lesions can safely be treated by partial nephrectomy in patients with a normal contralateral kidney. Patients who do not have a normal contralateral kidney are the best candidates for renal-sparing surgery. At the present time, open resection of the affected area of the kidney is the procedure of choice. As ureteroscopes and ureteroscopic instruments improve, the use of retrograde ureteropyeloscopy for the management of these tumors is likely to increase. Topical chemotherapy with thiotepa, mitomycin C, or BCG in the upper urinary tract may be of benefit for controlling recurrences following local resection [27]. The addition of adjuvent M-VAC chemotherapy also holds promise for improving survival in patients with this tumor.

References

1. Carini M, Selli C, Barbanti G, Lapini A, Turini D, Constantini A: Conservative surgical treatment of renal cell carcinoma: Clinical experience and reappraisal of indications. J Urol 140:725–731, 1988.
2. Schiff M Jr., Bagley D, Lytton B: Treatment of solitary and bilateral renal carcinomas. J Urol 121:581–583, 1979.

3. Graham S Jr., Glenn JF: Enucleative surgery for renal malignancy. J Urol 122:546–549, 1979.
4. Smith RB, DeKernion JB, Ehrlich RM, Skinner DG, Kaufman JJ: Bilateral renal cell carcinoma and renal cell carcinoma in the solitary kidney. J Urol 132:450–454, 1984.
5. Zincke H, Sen SE: Experience with extracorporeal surgery and autotransplantation for renal cell and transitional cell cancer of the kidney. J Urol 140:25–27, 1988.
6. Novick AC, Streem S, Montie JE, Pontes JE, Siegel S, Montague DK, Goormastic M: Conservative surgery for renal cell carcinoma: A single-center experience with 100 patients. J Urol 141:835–839, 1989.
7. Mukamel E, Konichezky M, Engelstein D, Servadio C: Incidental small renal tumors accompanying clinically overt renal cell carcinoma. J Urol 140:22–24, 1988.
8. Marshall FF, Taxy JB, Fishman EK, Chang R: The feasibility of surgical enucleation for renal cell carcinoma. J Urol 135:231–234, 1986.
9. Blackley SK, Ladaga L, Woolfitt RA, Schellhammer PF: Ex situ study of the effectiveness of enucleation in patients with renal cell carcinoma. J Urol 140:6–10, 1988.
10. Morgan WR, Zincke H: Progression and survival after renal-conserving surgery for renal cell carcinoma: Experience in 104 patients and extended followup. J Urol 144:852–858, 1990.
11. Talamo TS, Shonnard JW: Small renal adenocarcinoma with metastases. J Urol 124: 132–134, 1980.
12. DeKernion JB, Ramming KP, Smith RB: The natural history of metastatic renal cell carcinoma: A computer analysis. J Urol 120:148–152, 1978.
13. Takatera H, Maeda O, Oka T, Namiki M, Nakano E, Matsuda M, Arita N, Jamshidi J, Ushio Y, Sonoda T: Solitary late recurrence of renal cell carcinoma. J Urol 136:799–800, 1986.
14. Ljungberg B, Duchek M, Hietala S, Roos G, Stenling R: Renal cell carcinoma in a solitary kidney: Late nephrectomy after 35 years and analysis of tumor deoxyribonucleic acid content. J Urol 139:350–352, 1988.
15. Loughlin KR, Gittes RF: Urological management of patients with von Hippel-Lindau's disease. J Urol 136:789–791, 1986.
16. Malek RS, Omess PJ, Benson RC Jr., Zincke H: Renal cell carcinoma in von Hippel-Lindau syndrome. Am J Med 82:236–238, 1987.
17. Spencer WF, Novick AC, Montie JE, Streem SB, Levin HS: Surgical treatment of localized renal cell carcinoma in von Hippel-Lindau's disease. J Urol 139:507–509, 1988.
18. Calne RY: Tumour in a single kidney: Nephrectomy, excision and autotransplantation. Lancet 2:761, 1971.
19. Gelin L-E, Claes G, Gustafsson A, Storm B: Total bloodlessness for extracorporeal renal organ repair. Rev Surg 28:305, 1971.
20. Flatmark A, Sodal G, Jervel J. Brodwall E, Enge I: Preliminary experience with extracorporeal renal surgery and autotransplantation. Eur Surg Res 9:235, 1977.
21. Gittes RF, McCullough DL: Bench surgery for tumor in a solitary kidney. J Urol 113:12, 1975.
22. McLoughlin MG: The treatment of bilateral synchronous renal pelvic tumors with bench surgery. J Urol 114:463, 1975.
23. Hollabaugh RS, Cheek RC, Seller KD: A surgical approach to bilateral hypernephroma using "benchwork" excision and autotransplantation. Am Surg 42:411, 1976.
24. Kimball FN, Ferris HV: Papillomatous tumor of the renal pelvis associated with similar tumors of the ureter and bladder. A review of the literature and report of two cases. J Urol 31:257, 1934.
25. Gittes RF: Management of transitional cell carcinoma of the upper tract: Case for conservative local excision. Urol Clin North Am 7(3):559–568, 1980.
26. Blute ML, Segura JW, Patterson DE, Benson RC Jr., Zincke H: Impact of endourology on diagnosis and management of upper urinary tract urothelial cancer. J Urol 141:1298–1301, 1989.

27. Smith AD, Orihuela E, Crowley AR: Percutaneous management of renal pelvic tumors: A treatment option in selected cases. J Urol 137:852–856, 1987.
28. Huffman JL: Ureteroscopic management of transitional cell carcinoma of the upper urinary tract. Urol Clin North Am 15(3):419–424, 1988.
29. Murphy DM, Zincke H, Furlow WL: Primary grade 1 transitional cell carcinoma of the renal pelvis and ureter. J Urol 123:629–631, 1980.
30. Sternberg CA, Yagoda A, Scher HI, Watson RC, Herr HW, Morse MJ, Sogani RC, Vaughan ED Jr., Bander N, Weiselberg LR, Geller N, Hollander PH, Lipperman R, Fair WR, Whitmore WF Jr.: M-VAC (methotrexate, vinblastine, doxorubicin and cisplatin) for advanced transitional cell carcinoma of the urothelium. J Urol 139:461–469, 1988.
31. Wallace DMA, Wallace DM, Whitfield HN, Hendry WF, Wickham JEA: The late results of conservative surgery for upper tract urothelial carcinomas. Br J Urol 53:537–541, 1981.
32. Ziegelbaum M, Novick AC, Streem SB, Montie JE, Pontes JE, Straffon RA: Conservative surgery for transitional cell carcinoma of the renal pelvis. J Urol 138:1146–1149, 1987.
33. Faysel MH, Freiha FS: Evaluation of partial cystectomy for carcinoma of bladder. Urology 4(14):352–356, 1979.
34. Bagley DH: Flexible endoscopy in the urinary tract. Semin Urol 4:198, 1986.

3. A comparison of the treatment of metastatic prostate cancer by testicular ablation or total androgen blockade

The Canadian Anandron Study Group*

Background

In 1941 Huggins and Hodges discovered that prostatic cancer was androgen dependent [1,2]. They reasoned that if the normal prostate were androgen dependent, then prostatic cancer also should be similarly dependent, and that androgen deprivation should inhibit the growth of the tumor. This hypothesis was tested by many investigators in the hope that the gloomy prognosis associated with advanced prostatic cancer could be altered. Indeed, the dramatic responses initiated by castration or the administration of large doses of estrogens suggested to early investigators that this form of therapy might cure the disease. However, subsequent larger trials inevitably recorded that, while this therapy played a major palliative role, most patients with advanced prostatic cancer treated with hormonal ablation soon died of their disease [3,4]. This observation suggested that either the theory that the tumor was androgen dependent was not entirely true or that the method of achieving androgen deprivation was imperfect.

Brendler and others believed that the latter might be true. They initiated trials to eliminate the residual amount of adrenal androgen remaining after castration by surgical adrenalectomy or hypophysectomy in patients who had failed primary hormonal therapy. These early trials were fraught with severe complications, as the source and mechanisms of action of glucocorticoids were not well understood. The results of these trials using sequential forms of androgen deprivation failed to convince the investigators that this was an advantageous form of therapy [5]. Later large studies by the Veterans Administration Genito-Urinary Study Group suggested that hormonal therapy might have no survival benefit and its only use was palliative [6].

* Members of the study group include Dr. G. Beland, University of Montreal, Montreal, Quebec; Dr. M. Elhilali, McGill University, Montreal, Quebec; Dr. Y. Fradet and Dr. B. Laroche, Laval University, Quebec, Quebec; Dr. E. Ramsey, University of Manitoba, Winnipeg, Manitoba; Dr. J. Trachtenberg, University of Toronto, Toronto, Ontario; Dr. H. Tewari, St. John Regional Hospital, St. John, New Brunswick, and Dr. P. Venner, University of Alberta, Edmonton, Alberta.

Lepor, H. and Lawson R.K., (eds.), Therapy for Genitourinary Cancer. *ISBN 0-7923-1412-3.*

With the discovery of several pharmaceuticals that were potent competitive blockers of the intracellular androgen receptor, it became clinically possible to test the hypothesis of whether "total androgen blockade" (TAB), i.e., simultaneous elimination of testicular and adrenal androgen, might be that form of androgen deprivation that would finally prove the initial theory that failures of hormonal therapy were due to inadequate treatment. Several trials combined antiandrogens (either steroidal or nonsteroidal) and medical or surgical castration, and compared the duration of response and survival of this treatment in patients with metastatic prostatic cancer with similar patients treated by castration alone. The results, in general, suggested that there was little or no advantage to TAB [7,8]. In 1977 Bracci reported that orchiectomy combined with cyproterone acetate was superior to orchiectomy alone [9]. Labrie published that TAB effected by a nonsteroidal antiandrogen and a medical means of testicular ablation [luteinizing hormone releasing hormone (LHRH) agonist analogues] would cause a spectacular improvement in the duration of response and survival. Indeed, several claims suggested that this treatment was tantamount to "cure" [10,11]. No comparative trials were conducted by this group to prove their impressions.

Because of the enormous clinical implications of this finding, several large clinical trials were mounted to try to decide the exact benefit that TAB might effect. These trials have mirrored the questions that each group felt was pertinent at the moment that the trial was initiated. They also reflect the clinical feelings of the national origins of the groups and the availability of novel pharmaceuticals at the time of initiation of the trials.

The largest individual trial conducted to date attempted to determine the validity of the Labrie observations, namely, can the combination of an LHRH analogue and an antiandrogen improve the survival of patients with metastatic prostate cancer as compared to those patients treated by an LHRH analogue alone — a conventional form of testicular ablation [12]. This was a multicenter, placebo-controlled, double-blind randomized trial that began in 1985 and was sponsored by the National Cancer Institute of the National Institutes of Health. Six hundred and three men with stage D2 prostate cancer were randomized to treatment with either daily subcutaneous injections of leuprolide (an LHRH agonist analogue, Lupron), and a placebo or leuprolide, and the nonsteroidal antiandrogen flutamide (Eulexin). The 303 men receiving androgen blockade with leuprolide and flutamide demonstrated a longer progression-free survival (16.9 vs. 13.9 months, $p = 0.039$) and an increased median length of survival (35.0 vs. 27.9 months, $p = 0.035$). In the subgroup of men with minimal disease and good performance status, the advantages of maximal androgen blockade appeared pronounced. These investigators concluded that combined androgen blockade with leuprolide and flutamide was superior to treatment with leuprolide alone.

Two European trials have also attempted to answer this question. They have been reported individually and with their data pooled. The Urologic

Group of the European Organization on Research and Treatment of Cancer (EORTC) compared the outcome of therapy of 327 men with metastatic prostate cancer treated with either Zoladex (a long-acting depot form of an LHRH agonist analogue) and the antiandrogen flutamide or bilateral orchiectomy [13]. The trial that began in 1986 (study 30853) noted a statistically significant increase in the time to subjective and objective progression in favor of the combination treatment. No differences were noted in the time to death by cancer or death by any cause.

A second similar trial was conducted independently by the Danish Prostate Cancer Group (DAPROCA) [14]. They randomized 264 patients with advanced prostate cancer to Zoladex and flutamide, or bilateral orchiectomy. After a median follow-up of 30 months, a difference in objective response was noted in favor of the combination, but no differences were noted in the time to progression and overall survival.

These two groups have pooled their data because of the similar nature and conduct of their studies. In doing so they have increased the power of the study to detect smaller but still significant treatment differences. In addition, they noted a small but significant difference in the time to objective progression or death from prostate cancer in favor of the combination therapy. However, the time from objective progression to death was longer in the group allocated to orchiectomy, and the overall survival was similar in the two groups. These authors thus concluded that combined androgen blockade was not superior to orchiectomy in the treatment of advanced prostate cancer [15].

The results of these trials are paradoxical and conflicting. While they all suggest that there may be some effect of TAB, the degree of this outcome varies from minimal (with little clinical benefit) to the possibility of many years of increased survival in appropriately chosen patients.

In 1984 we began a trial with a similar goal. In order to determine if combined androgen therapy might yield a significant improvement in the treatment of advanced prostatic cancer, we conducted a double-blind, prospective randomized trial of the form of TAB, castration, and a nonsteroidal pure antiandrogen (C-A) with castration. The preliminary results have been previously reported [16]. The final analysis of the 6 years of follow-up of these patients is presented in this report.

Methods

Two hundred and fifty-four patients with histologically documented metastatic prostatic cancer and without prior hormone or chemo therapy were screened at seven university teaching hospitals in Canada for entry to this trial. Informed consent was obtained from 208 patients before treatment, and they were then randomly assigned to either castration and placebo (group 1), or castration and the nonsteroidal pure antiandrogen, anandron

(Nilutimide, Roussel Pharmaceutical Inc., Montreal, Canada) at 100 mg po three times per day (C-A, group 2). This phase of the trial was double blinded. An open parallel trial was also conducted in the manner suggested by Labrie with the remaining 46 patients who refused orchiectomy [10]. These patients were treated with the luteinizing hormone releasing hormone (LHRH) agonist analogue Buserelin (Hoechst Pharmaceuticals, Montreal, Canada; 0.50 mg sc per day for 30 days then 0.25 mg sc per day) and also the antiandrogen Anandron in the dose described above (group 3). These patients were independently followed on the same follow-up protocol as those patients in the randomized trial described above. No statistical comparisons were performed between the first two groups and group 3.

Follow-up visits were on inclusion and after 1, 3, 6, and 12 months of treatment and every 3 months after that. At these encounters patients were subjected to extensive evaluations that included performance measurements (ECOG performance scale), pain rating (0–4), analgesic intake, voiding symptoms, and side effects. In addition, physical examinations with specific attention to the primary tumor were done. This was confirmed by transabdominal or transrectal ultrasonography. Routine biochemical and hematologic parameters were also obtained. Serum prostatic acid phosphatase, alkaline phosphatase, and testosterone were obtained at each visit. At 6-month intervals bone scans were repeated. The patients' responses were graded by the criteria of the National Prostatic Cancer Project. If a patient demonstrated objective evidence of progression, the code was broken and the patient was administered the antiandrogen if he was receiving the placebo. All patients were followed to death.

Two hundred and fifty-four patients were initially included in this study (103, 105, and 46 patients for groups 1, 2, and 3, respectively). The patients in groups 1 and 2 were subjected to a balanced randomization at each center. Nineteen patients were excluded from the study; seven because of incorrect staging, nine due to previous hormone therapy, and three due to a delay of >3 months in the administration of the antiandrogen. The percentage and type of exclusions were similar in each group, i.e., group 1, 7 patients (7%); group 2, 7 patients (7%); and group 3, 5 patients (11%). Ninety-six patients were thus in group 1, 98 in group 2, and 41 in group 3. These patients have now been followed for 36–72 months.

Statistical considerations

End points of the study were quality of life parameters (pain, analgesic consumption, performance status), "best response to treatment," time to progression, and survival. All statistical considerations were based only on groups 1 and 2. Statistical significance was judged at the $p < 0.05$ level. Changes in the severity of symptoms were analyzed by the Wilcoxon test. The best response to treatment was analyzed by a chi-squared analysis. The time to progression and death were estimated by the Kaplan Meier technique and compared by a log-rank evaluation. These assessments were performed on the statistical software package SAS run on an IBM 3083 computer.

Results

Entry characteristics

The median age of the patients on entry in groups 1, 2, and 3 were 69 (range, 42–90), 70 (range 47–93), and 65 (range 46–83), respectively. One hundred and thirty-three (59%) had moderate or severe bone pain on entry: 49 (53%), 58 (62%), and 26 (63%) in groups 1, 2, and 3, respectively. One hundred and thirty-six patients (60%) had an impaired performance status on entry: 55 (59%), 57 (62%), and 24 (56%) in groups 1, 2, and 3, respectively. One hundred and eighty-three patients (82%) had an elevated PAP on entry: 72 (82%) in group 1, 72 (80%) in group 2, and 23 (60%) in group 3. There were no statistically significant differences between groups 1 and 2 in any of the above parameters.

End points

Pain. In patients with bone pain on entry to the trial, no differences in "improvement" were noted between groups 1 and 2 at months 1 and 3. At 6 months, however, a significant difference was noted in favor of group 2 ($p = 0.003$). This should be contrasted with the results of the tracking of analgesic use in the groups at the same intervals. No differences in analgesic use was discernible between the two groups at any time.

Performance status. When all patients in groups 1 and 2 were considered, no significant differences in performance status at any point between the two groups was noted. In patients with impaired performance status on entry, the difference in the degree of improvement of performance during treatment between groups 1 and 2 was never significant.

Biochemical parameters

Serum prostatic acid phosphatase did not demonstrate a significant difference in group 2 as compared to group 1 at any time point. In contrast, measurements of serum alkaline phosphatase did demonstrate significant changes between groups 1 and 2 at month 3 ($p = 0.002$) and month 6 ($p < 0.001$), but not at month 1 ($p = 0.18$). None of the other biochemical parameters measured demonstrated any significant difference between the two evaluated groups at any time point.

Best response to treatment

Whether "stable" disease was considered as a response to treatment or not, the percentage of responses was significantly higher in group 2 than in group 1. In the first case (response = complete regression + partial regression + stable), the percentage of responders was 61% in group 1 and 78% in group 2 ($p = 0.013$); in the second case (response = complete regression + partial regression), the percentage of responders was 20% in group 1 and 45% in group 2 ($p < 0.001$). Patients in group 3 responded similarly to those of group 2.

Time to progression

There was no significant difference in the time to progression in the two comparison groups (Figure 1; $p = 0.462$). The progression-free actuarial rate at 6, 12, 18, and 24 months for groups 1 and 2 were 65%, 47%, 27%, and 21% vs. 80%, 53%, 39%, and 22%, respectively. These values were not significantly different. The median time to progression was 11.7 and 12.4 months in groups 1 and 2, respectively. These values are not significantly different.

Time to death

The time to death from cancer (Figure 2) or the time to death from all causes (Figure 3) was not significantly longer in group 2 than in group 1. The

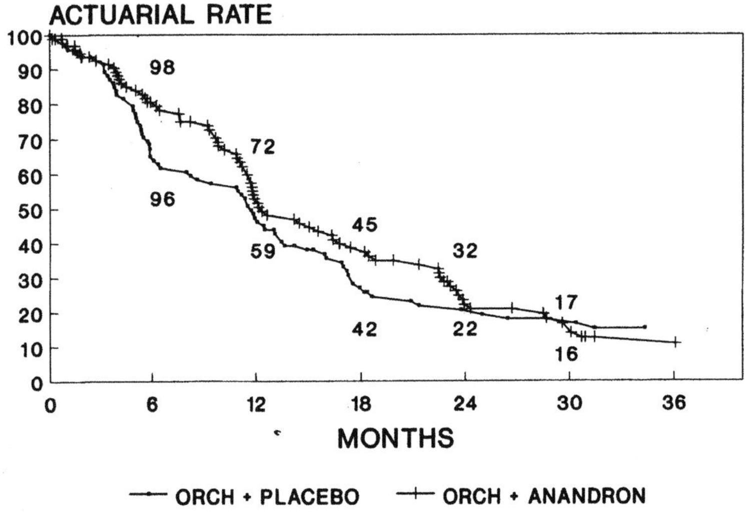

Figure 1. The actuarial rate of progression of patients treated with castration and Anandron (++++) or castration and placebo (----); log rank evaluation, $p = 0.462$.

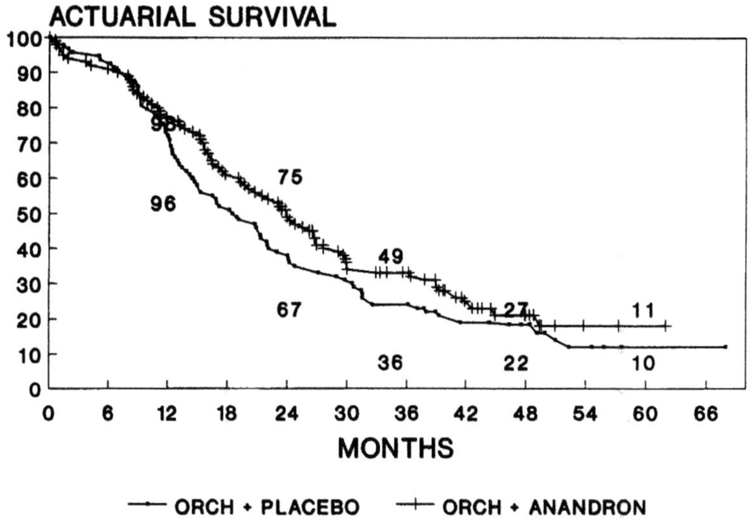

Figure 2. The actuarial rate of survival (death due to cancer) of patients treated with castration and Anandron (++++) or castration and placebo (----); log rank evaluation, p = 0.181.

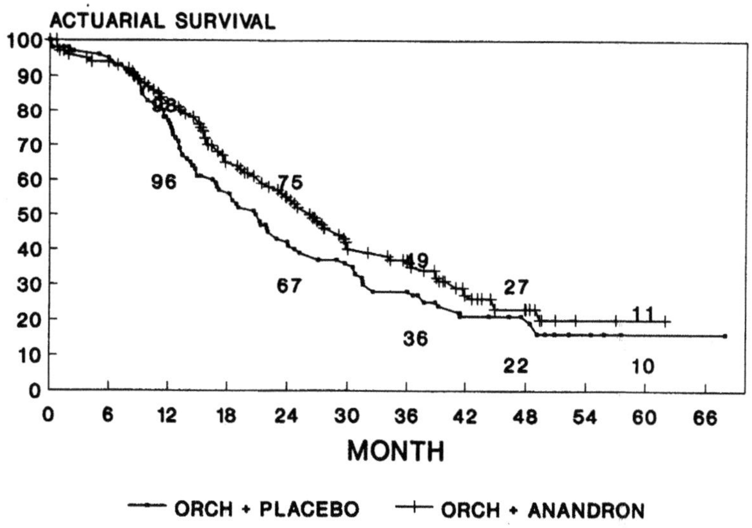

Figure 3. The actuarial rate of survival (death due to all causes) of patients treated with castration and Anandron (++++) or castration and placebo (----); log rank evaluation, p = 0.137.

median survival of group 1 was 21.2 months vs. 26.5 months in group 2 when death due to cancer was considered and 18.9 vs. 24.3 months when death due to any cause was calculated. The log-rank analysis yielded a p value of 0.181 in the former case and a p value of 0.137 in the latter case.

Table 1. Adverse effects of treatment

Adverse Effects	Castration + Placebo (n = 97[a])	Castration + Nilutamide (n = 99[a])
Minor		
Hot flashes	65 (67%)	76 (77%)
Impaired adaption to darkness	14 (14%)	40 (40%)
Alcohol intolerance	6 (6%)	17 (17%)
Nausea	6 (6%)	13 (13%)[b]
Major (necessitating discontinuation of therapy)		
Dizziness and headaches	0	1
Nausea	1	0
Interstitial pneumonitis	0	2
Visual problems	0	1
Pruritus	0	1
Increased liver enzymes	0	1
Hot flushes	0	3[c]
Total	1 (1%)	9 (9%)

[a] Tolerance was not evaluable for 5 patients in the placebo group and for 2 patients in the nilutamide group because they either never took the medication or received it for less than one month.

[b] Nilutamide tolerated with decreased dose in 4 patients.

[c] Two patients with hot flushes had concomitant progression of their disease when they were discontinued.

Adverse effects

Loss of libido and impotence were commonly found in both groups. Hot flashes was the most frequent adverse effect encountered during this study, and the frequency was not significantly different for the two groups. There were significantly more adverse effects in group 2 than in group 1 ($p = 0.040$). Although these were largely minor in nature and were related to visual (impaired dark adaptability) and gastrointestinal (alcohol intolerance and nausea) causes, several patients had severe side effects that necessitated a change in the study protocol (Table 1). Nausea and vomiting forced a decrease in Anandron dosage in four patients. Anandron was stopped in three patients for hot flashes, in two patients for interstitial lung disease, and in one patient each for a visual problem, pruritus, dizziness/headaches, and increased liver enzymes. No patient had a fatal complication of therapy, and all ill effects were reversible on altering the dose of the antiandrogen or on stopping treatment. One patient had his treatment permanently stoped due to adverse effects in group 1, while nine patients had their treatment discontinued due to adverse effects in group 2. The rate of clinically important side effects necessitating a temporary or permanent change of therapy was significantly higher in group 2. Thus, thirteen percent of patients had their treatment altered in group 2 as opposed to only 1% in group 1.

Discussion

Since the initiation of the treatment of advanced prostate cancer by androgen ablation in 1941, no significant increase in survival has been noted with this therapy. Labrie's studies noting a marked increase in the time to progression and survival by combined hormonal therapy suggested that the failure of hormonal therapy might have been the result of inadequate androgen blockade and not a failure of the concept of substantial androgen dependence of prostate cancer [10,11]. The present study compared the outcome of patients with metastatic prostatic cancer treated with either castration or castration and an antiandrogen — a form of "total androgen ablation." In essence, it attempted to demonstrate whether the addition of an antiandrogen to castration would yield improved results. The choice of surgical castration as the standard arm of therapy was crucial in the design of this trial. Although the studies reported by Labrie used an LHRH analogue agonist for medical castration that was then combined with antiandrogen therapy, we believe that LHRH analogue therapy alone does not lend itself well for use as the control arm of a study of total androgen blockade. This conclusion is based on the well-documented occurrence of an increase of serum testosterone in the first weeks of administration of this drug. This is often accompanied by a temporary deterioration in the patient's symptoms, which then improve when the paradoxical suppression of testosterone production comes into play [17]. Thus a comparison of an LHRH analogue agonist alone and an LHRH analogue agonist plus an antiandrogen might be expected to yield improved early results in the combination group merely because of suppression of the iatrogenic-induced temporary deterioration caused by use of the LHRH analogue alone. No antitumor effect of therapy thus would necessarily be demonstrated. Results of the Intergroup trial sponsored by the National Cancer Institute showing benefit to combination therapy have been justly criticized on such a basis [12]. The results of the European trials cited above failed to demonstrate as great an advantage to TAB compared an LHRH analogue agonist and an antiandrogen against castration [13–15]. One could speculate from comparing the results of these trial that perhaps the effectiveness of the two control arms are not exactly equivalent. Indeed, the investigators of the Intergroup trial have now embarked on a large trial of castration vs. castration and an antiandrogen to see if they can achieve a similar outcome with this protocol as their initial study.

The results of the study described in this paper represent the final analysis of our trial. They illustrate the difficulties in the conduct of any trial dealing with the treatment of metastatic prostatic cancer. These problems have been amply elaborated on by many authors, but include the lack of truly objective measuring instruments, the fluctuating nature of many so-called tumor markers, the propensity to use subjective measuring instruments, the inadequate schemes of measuring response, and of most importance, the variable natural history of the disease. Nonetheless, we believe that the questions posed by total androgen ablation in the treatment of metastatic prostatic cancer justified the execution of the above trial, in spite of its inherent difficulties.

The results of this trial suggest that total androgen ablation may offer an advantage in the treatment of advanced prostatic cancer. The exact nature of this advantage must be carefully analyzed to derive reasonable clinical guidelines for the treatment of metastatic prostatic cancer. This study was initiated in response to the spectacular results claimed by Labrie. He and his colleagues claimed that the combination of an LHRH analogue agonist and the antiandrogen Anandron resulted in >80% 2-year survival and >60% 2-year disease-free survival in a study of 119 patients with metastatic prostatic cancer [10]. Clearly these results were not duplicated in this trial or any of the above-mentioned trials. Also, the extent of improvement over conventional treatment realized in this trial, although important and statistically significant, is not spectacular. In addition, these gains were obtained only with an increased incidence of adverse effects that, although mild in most cases, were life threatening in a few patients (those patients with interstitial pneumonitis).

The clearest outcome of the present trial was that the group of patients treated with combined therapy showed a greater number of responders than did the conventionally treated group. This finding held true whether the category of "stable" was included or excluded as a response. The importance of this observation must be tempered with the fact that the response, no matter how great, did not seem to last dramatically long. In addition, classical measures of improvement of quality of life, such as pain, analgesic use, or performance status, did not show consistent improvement throughout the treatment period.

The result of the actuarial analysis of the time to progression did not show any difference between the two treatment arms and demonstrated a similar median time to progression. Since most patients eventually died while on treatment, any benefit derived from C-A would be expected to arise early in the course of therapy. We have reanalyzed the time to progression using the Wilcoxon test. As opposed to the log-rank analysis, which equally weighs all aspects of the actuarial curve, the Wilcoxon analysis stresses the initial phases of the curve. Even using this method, a significant difference in the time to progression curves was not found in favor of the C-A group ($p = 0.152$). The progression-free actuarial rates were similar in the two groups at 12 or more months (47% vs. 53% at month 12, 27% vs. 39% at month 18, and 21% vs. 22% at month 24 for the placebo group and the C-A group, respectively).

There was not a statistically significant advantage in favor of the combined treatment group in terms of overall survival, although a 5- to 6-month trend toward increased survival was noted. These data suggest that if there is a difference in the time to death, the power of this study to demonstrate it may be limited by the small patient population. Further calculations have suggested that similar results with a patient population approximately 30% larger would yield statistical significance. Although the difference of 6 months was not spectacular, it nonetheless does represent a 33% increase in survival over the control group.

The difference in the median survival between the two groups was approximately 6 months. Since the conduct of this trial was of a crossover variety, all patients received the antiandrogen from the time of progression until death. Thus the only difference in the treatment of these patients was in the period from the initiation of therapy to progression. It thus would appear that the maximal benefit of C-A occurs only with the concomitant administration of the two modalities of androgen ablation at the initiation of therapy. Conversely, one might speculate that delayed (at progression) administration of the antiandrogen did not confer a significant benefit to the patients who were initially treated with the placebo.

There was a significantly increased incidence of side effects in the C-A group. However, most of these side effects were mild, tolerable, or reversible. Liver and pulmonary function should be monitored and treatment should be altered if signs of dysfunction appear. Since the advantages of C-A in terms of quality of response and possibly duration of survival may be real, the drug-related difficulties encountered appear to be a price most patients would be willing to pay.

The results of this trial suggest that certain patients derive significant benefit from total androgen ablation in the treatment of advanced prostatic cancer. Other studies have suggested that patients with minimal tumor burden are maximally helped by TAB [12]. Unfortunately, the patient population in this study is too small to allow for adequate substratification, and therefore, confirmation of the above observation.

The ultimate goal of this and other trials is to uncover the degree of benefit afforded by TAB and which patients gain the most from this form of treatment. An attempt to conduct a meta-analysis to answer these questions has been proposed by Dr. L. Denis of the EORTC and is being pursued with the support of this agency and the American Cancer Society [18]. When this study is accomplished, the above questions should be answered.

Nonetheless, this and other studies of TAB have still demonstrated a median survival of less than 3.5 years for all patients with metastatic prostate cancer. Thus the overall outlook for patients with this form of advanced cancer remains gloomy, no matter what type of hormonal manipulation is performed. The cure of this disease lies in other avenues of treatment.

Acknowledgments

Supported in part by a grant from Roussel Pharmaceuticals, Canada. The authors wish to acknowledge the encouragement and generous support of

Dr. J. Gareau and Roussel Pharmaceuticals Canada in the conduct of this study.

References

1. Huggins C, Hodges CV: Studies on prostatic cancer: 1. The effect of castration, of estrogen and of androgen injection on serum phosphatases in metastatic carcinoma of the prostate. Cancer Res 11:293, 1941.
2. Huggins C, Stevens RE, Hodges CV: Studies on prostatic cancer: II The effects of castration on advanced carcinoma of the prostate gland. Arch Surg 43:209, 1941.
3. Lepor H, Ross A, Walsh PC: The influence of hormonal therapy on survival of men with advanced prostatic cancer. J Urolo 128:335, 1982.
4. Vest SA, Frazier TH: Survival following castration for prostatic cancer. J Urol 56:97, 1946.
5. Brendler H: Adrenalectomy and hypophysectomy for prostatic cancer. Urology 2:99, 1973.
6. Veterans Administration Cooperative Urological Research Group: Treatment and survival of patients with cancer of the prostate. Surg Gynecol Obstet 124:1011, 1967.
7. Schroeder FH, Klijn JG, de Jong FH: Metastatic cancer of the prostate managed by Buserelin acetate verus Buserelin acetate plus cyproterone acetate. Proceedings of the Annual Meeting of the American Urological Association, New York, 1986.
8. Denis L, DeMoura C, Smith P, et al.: Zoladex and Flutamide verus orchiectomy: First final analysis of EORTC 30853. Proceedings of the Annual Meeting of the American Urological Association, Dallas, 1989.
9. Bracci U: Present procedures in the treatment of prostate cancer. In: Bracci U, Di Silverio F (eds). *Hormonal Therapy of Prostate Cancer*. Cofese, Palermo, 1977, pp. 744–750.
10. Labrie F, Dupont A, Belanger A, Cusan L, Lacourciere Y, Monfette G, Laberge JG, Emond JP, Fazekas ATA, Raynaud JP, Husson JM: New hormonal therapy in prostatic cancer: Combined treatment with an LHRH agonist and an antiandrogen. Clin Invest Med 5:267, 1982.
11. Labrie F, Dupont A, Belanger A, Cusan L, Lacourciere Y, Emond JP, Monfette G, Laberge JG, Bergeron B, Harnois C: Antiandrogens and LHRH agonists in the treatment of prostatic cancer. Medicine/Science 1:435, 1985.
12. Crawford ED, Eisenberger MA, McLeod DG, Spaulding JT, Benson R, Dorr FA, Blumenstein BA, Davis MA, Goodman PJ: A controlled trial of leuprolide with and without flutamide in prostatic carcinoma. N Engl J Med 321(7):419–424, 1989.
13. Iversen P, Christensen MG, Friis F, et al.: A phase 111 trial of Zoladex and Flutamide versus orchiectomy in the treatment of patients with advanced carcinoma of the prostate. Cancer 66(5) (Suppl.):52–69, 1990.
14. Keuppens F, Denis L, Smith P, et al.: Zoladex and Flutamide versus bilateral orchiectomy. Cancer 66(5) (Suppl.):39–51, 1990.
15. Iversen P, Suciu S, Sylvester R, et al. Zoladex and Flutamide versus orchiectomy in the treatment of advanced prostate cancer. Cancer 66(5) (Suppl.):61–67, 1990.
16. Beland J, Elhilali M, Fradet Y, et al.: A prospective randomized trial of castration and Anandron vs castration and placebo in metastatic prostatic cancer. Proceedings of the Annual Meeting of the Canadian Urologic Association, Banff, Alberta, 1987.
17. The Leuprolide Study Group: Leuprolide vs. DES in the initial therapy of advanced prostatic cancer: A randomized prospective trial. N Engl J Med 311(20):1281, 1984.
18. Dalesio O. Complete androgen blockade in prostate cancer. Cancer 66(5) (Suppl.):74–76, 1990.

4. The role of radiotherapy following radical prostatectomy

Michael K. Brawer

Adenocarcinoma of the prostate is currently the number one malignancy in men in the United States and the second most common cause of cancer-related deaths [1]. In part because of these sobering statistics, there has been increasing interest in curative therapy. Radical prostatectomy is emerging as the preferred therapeutic approach for a number of reasons. If neoplasm is organ confined, surgical extirpation offers the best chance of cure. Moreover, increasing evidence suggests that definitive radiation therapy is rarely able to sterilize the prostate [2]. Finally, technical advances have made radical retropubic prostatectomy more acceptable because of decreased morbidity.

Unfortunately, a high percentage of patients, despite clinical assessment indicating organ-confined disease, have extension beyond the confines of the prostate (pathologic upstaging). Radiation therapy following radical prostatectomy has been advocated as a means of providing adjuvant treatment to those patients who have an increased likelihood of local or distant failure. In this chapter we will discuss the role of radiation therapy following radical prostatectomy. The high incidence of surgical upstaging will be reviewed, along with the current limitations of imaging modalities to predict cancer extension preoperatively. Methods of assessment of persistent disease will be reviewed, and the results of adjuvant radiation therapy trials will be discussed.

Virtually every series on radical prostatectomy demonstrates significant pathologic upstaging of what was felt to be clinically localized disease. Table 1 reviews several series [3–8]. This upstaging occurs in 11–50% of men with clinical stage A carcinoma, 17–25% of those with B_1, and 39–68% of those with clinical B_2 prostate cancer.

The digital rectal examination is woefully inadequate in the assessment of tumor extent. For example, Spigelman and associates demonstrated 7 of 17 patients had a tumor volume at the time of radical prostatectomy of more than twice that estimated preoperatively based on digital rectal examination [9].

Unfortunately, modern imaging modalities offer little advantage over the digital rectal examination preoperative assessment of the pathologic stage.

Lepor, H. and Lawson R.K., (eds.), Therapy for Genitourinary Cancer.
Kluwer Academic Publishers. ISBN 0-7923-1412-3.

Table 1. Incidence of extracapsular disease after radical prostatectomy

Clinical Author	Reference	Stage	Number	Upstaged (%)
Lange	3	A2	6	3 (50)
Catalona	4	A2	9	1 (11)
Veenema	5	A, B	159	66 (42)
Jewett	6	B1	103	26 (25)
Catalona	4	B1	48	8 (17)
Gibbons	7	B	143	46 (31)
Lange	3	B2	25	15 (60)
Catalona	4	B2	23	9 (39)
Elder	8	B2	53	35 (66)

Computer-assisted tomography has been well studied in this regard, and most authors conclude that it is inadequate in providing useful information for local staging. Recently there has been increased interest in magnetic resonance imaging with regard to local staging. While some authorities have suggested this modality provides a significant improvement over CT, more information will be necessary before meaningful conclusions can be drawn as to the role of this technique in staging.

Transrectal ultrasound is felt by many authorities to represent the current best imaging modality for the prostate. Despite its usefulness in guiding transrectal biopsies, the application of this technology for staging remains largely unproven [10].

Several authors have attempted to correlate the sonographic findings with pathologic reconstructions of the surgical prostatectomy specimen [11–14]. While various criteria have been developed for the ultrasound characteristics of capsular penetration, positive margins, and seminal vesicle invasion, the accuracy seems to be largely operator dependent, and a significant incidence of false-positive and -negative scans occur. Lee has recommended ultrasound-guided biopsy for staging [15]. He has called particular attention to two sites of anatomic weakness: the so-called trapezoid space at the prostatic apex and the invaginated extra-prostatic space accompanying the ejaculatory ducts. While the sonographic appearance of tumor broaching the prostatic capsule may be nebulous, despite careful scrutiny with ultrasound of these areas, it is possible to guide the biopsy needle into these sites or into the seminal vesicles and to prove histologically extracapsular disease.

Prostate-specific antigen represents a major advance in our tumor-marker armamentarium. The complete organ specificity of this analyte makes it particularly useful in monitoring patients following radical prostatectomy. PSA has been examined with regard to its ability to predict the pathologic stage. Figure 1 illustrates the preoperative PSA in a personal radical prostatectomy series in which step-sectioning perpendicular to the rectal surface was performed on the surgical specimens. Note that while there is a correlation between PSA value and pathologic stage among the population as a

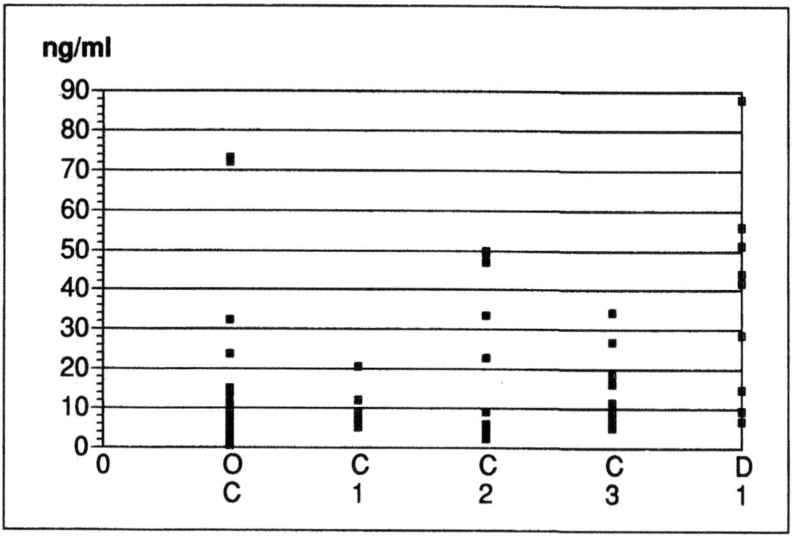

Figure 1. Preoperative prostate-specific antigen (PSA) (Tandem-R, Hybritech, San Diego, CA) and pathologic stage. OC = indicates organ-confined neoplasm; C1 = capsular penetration; C2 = capsular perforation; C3 = seminal vesicle invasion; D1 = pelvic lymph node metastases.

whole, significant overlap within any pathological stage obviates the discriminatory value for this assay in an individual patient. While a high preoperative PSA is generally a poor prognostic sign, no upper limit cutoff can be determined with which one could reliably exclude a significant number of people from radical surgery because of the possibility of false-positive values.

A final note with regard to preoperative staging is perhaps in order. Staging is meaningful only in as much as it alters the course of therapy. Little patient benefit is derived from such technical advances as magnetic resonance imaging, staging transrectal ultrasound biopsy, or laparoscopic assessment of the pelvic lymph nodes if these do not modify the planned therapeutic approach. Until data are available that definitively assess the role of these modalities, a carefully performed digitally rectal examination and bone scan remain the most important preoperative staging tests.

The thoroughness of the pathologic assessment of the surgical specimen is obviously of extreme importance. Clearly, if only one or two random specimens are taken through the prostate and seminal vesicles, the likelihood of detecting advanced local disease is lessened. The Stanford group has emphasized the importance of careful histologic reconstruction of the prostate with detailed scrutiny of the surgical margins [16]. Only with such attention to detail can the true pathologic stage be assessed. Several authors have subdivided stage C disease based on the level of capsular penetration and the presence of seminal vesicle extension, and have correlated this with prognostic importance [3,17–20].

Another factor of importance when comparing series is whether or not pelvic lymph node dissection was performed and whether frozen sections were included. This is the result of the stage migration phenomena that may occur if series where pelvic lymph node dissection is performed are compared to ones where either no pelvic lymph node dissection is performed or the thoroughness of the lymphadenectomy is not equivalent. Stage migration assumes that the local stage is lower in patients who have extensive examination of the pelvic lymph node, because patients with metastatic disease may not have been included in the radical prostatectomy series. Moreover, if frozen sections are included, microscopic metastatic disease may be appreciated and thus the pathologic differences between series with and without node dissection may be heightened.

Evidence of persistent disease

Perhaps the most accurate evidence indicating persistent carcinoma is that derived from the pathologic examination of the surgical specimen. If the margins are positive, one can generally conclude that cancer has been left behind. Again, the compulsiveness of the surgical pathologist's study of the specimen is obviously of great importance. More recently however, this concept has been called into some question. While most authorities consider tumor cells on the ink margin as evidence of disease left behind, others have cast doubt on the significance of this [21]. Clearly a long-term follow-up of patients who have had careful analysis of surgical specimens is necessary before we can know what the real impact of microscopic capsular penetration or perforation is.

Classically local occurrence has been diagnosed by an abnormal digital rectal examination. The accuracy of digital rectal examination in predicting carcinoma has only recently been addressed. Lange and associates have performed digitally guided needle biopsies of the region of the vesicle urethral anastomosis in 89 men following radical prostatectomy [22]. Among 57 men who had an elevated PSA, an average of 36 months following radical prostatectomy, they noted carcinoma in 42%. None of the 32 men who had nondetectable PSA was shown to be positive. These authors showed little relationship between the degree of palpable abnormality and the presence of carcinoma.

Recently we have utilized transrectal ultrasound in a number of men following radical prostatectomy to evaluate local disease persistence. Our most common observations in men with persistent disease are hypoechoic lesions adjacent to the vesical urethral anastamosis. Whether this modality will improve our ability to detect local recurrence remains to be proven.

Utilizing metastatic prostatic carcinoma, as evidenced by radionucleotide bone scan or other imaging modalities, to assess the utility of adjuvant therapy following radical prostatectomy is problematic. While obviously metastatic disease signifies disease persistence, it is not possible to resolve whether the metastases occurred prior to surgery but were present in such a low volume as to be undetectable by preoperative staging studies, or whether metastases resulted from neoplasm remaining at the surgical site.

Following radical prostatectomy, any PSA value higher than the lowest level of detectability is significant. This lower level of detectability must be ascertained in each laboratory. Lange and associates have demonstrated that a PSA >0.4 utilizing the Hybritech Tandem-R test is significant [23]. For example, these authors reported that disease occurred in all men who had a PSA >0.4 mg/ml, but in only 8% of those who had a PSA 3 or more months following radical prostatectomy of <0.2 nm/ml.

Despite the reliability of detectable PSA follow radical prostatectomy, the site of the neoplasm remains unknown. While local disease persistence may well be the cause of the abnormal test, equally likely is subclinical metastatic deposits [24].

One problem with PSA is that the current assays may not be sensitive enough to detect small-volume persistent disease. It is not uncommon to have a PSA level following radical prostatectomy that falls to the nondetectable level and remains there for several months to years, only then to begin to rise. Such observations clearly suggest a lack of a sensitivity of the assay. In an effort to obviate this problem, several laboratories are trying to develop a more sensitive PSA assay.

Results of radical prostatectomy alone

Before an analysis of the effect of adjuvant radiation therapy can be performed, one must be aware of the results of radical prostatectomy alone in the treatment of prostatic carcinoma. Table 2 demonstrates data from three studies of patients followed >15 years [6–8]. It is important to note that in these reports endocrine manipulation was not given until documentation of disease progression, with the exception of a few patients receiving a short course of perioperative hormonal manipulation. Jewett reported that 33% of these patients had no evidence of disease recurrence 15 years or more

Table 2. Radical prostatectomy 15-year NED[a] survival

Author	Reference	Clinical Stage	Pathologic Stage	No.	15-Year NED Survival (%)
Jewett	6	B1	B-C2	86	28 (33)
			C3	17	0
Gibbons	7	B1	B,C	43	26 (61)
		B2	B,C	9	3 (33)
Elder	8	B2	B	14	7 (50)
			C2-3	32	4 (13)

[a] NED = no evidence of disease.

Table 3. Pelvic disease persistence after radical prostatectomy

Pathologic Stage	References	Number of Pts.	Recurrence (%)
B	7,25,26	222	10–26
C	7,19,27–29	77	8–31
D_1	19,31	76	11–25

following radical prostatectomy [6]. Of note, none of his patients with seminal vesicle disease were without evidence of disease in 15 years. Elder and colleagues, reporting a subsequent series from the Johns Hopkins Hospital, reported 50% 15-year disease-free survival in patients with pathologically organ-confined disease, contrasting with a 13% disease-free status in those with capsular penetration and seminal vesicle invasion [8]. Gibbons and associates at the Mason Clinic described 43 patients with clinical B_1 disease followed for at least 15 years [7]. In 61% of their patients there was no evidence of disease at the latest follow-up. Only 3 of 9 patients with clinical B_2 disease were without evidence of persistence. It must be emphasized that these investigators utilized perineal prostatectomy, and pelvic lymph-node dissection was rarely performed. Nevertheless, these represent the series with the longest follow-up and must be utilized to compare adjuvant radiation therapy series.

Because of the impossibility of determining whether metastatic lesions were present at the time of radical prostatectomy, carcinoma persistence following radical prostatectomy is best discussed with regard to local disease. Several authors have assessed persistent pelvic malignancy following radical prostatectomy, and these are depicted in Table 3 [7,19,25–31]. In these series, adjuvant endocrine manipulation was withheld until disease persistence was documented. Local recurrence correlates strongly with pathologic stage and may be expected in 10–20% of organ-confined cancer, 8–31% of stage C disease, and 11–28% of those with pelvic lymph-node metastases.

Most authors report data indicating improved local recurrence rates in men receiving adjuvant radiation therapy for advanced local disease. For instance, whereas local recurrence was identified in a compilation of series in 32 of 291 (17%) men with pathologic stage C disease receiving radical prostatectomy alone (Table 3), only 6% (10 of 174) of patients had recurrence following radical prostatectomy and radiation therapy in Stage C and D1 disease (Table 4) [32–39].

Two authors have reported intra-institutional series in which patients receiving no adjuvant after radical prostatectomy were compared with an adjuvant radiation population [33,36]. It must be emphasized that these were not randomized studies, and the indications for administration of adjuvant therapy were not standardized. These authors described local recurrence rates in 0–5% of patients receiving adjuvant radiation therapy, as compared to 17–30% of those who did not.

Table 4. Pelvic disease persistence after radical prostatectomy and adjuvant radiation therapy

Pathologic Stage	References	Number of Pts.	Recurrence (%)
B	32	34	3
C	7,32,34–37	135	0–23
D_1	32,34,37	54	3–17

Table 5. Disease free survival following radical prostatectomy with adjuvant radiation therapy

Pathologic Stage	Reference	Number of Pts.	5-Year Disease Free (%)
B	32	34	88
C	7,32,34–37	135	57–80
D_1	32,34,37	54	41–92

One difficulty in evaluating the effectiveness of external beam radiation therapy in an adjuvant mode is that the length of follow-up in these reports is short. Despite these limitations, it is generally accepted that adjuvant external-beam radiation therapy is associated with decreased local disease persistence, at least as evidenced by digital rectal examination.

The ability of adjuvant radiation therapy to improve survival is even less well demonstrated. Table 5 depicts the disease-free survival in several reports. As shown in these series, the 5-year disease-free survival for stage C disease treated with adjuvant radiation therapy was between 65% and 80%, and in D-1 disease it was 41–92% [32–38]. A comparison with Table 1 shows that these figures are similar to the long-term follow-up of patients with organ-confined disease treated with radical prostatectomy alone. However, it is important to note that the length of follow-up in the adjuvant radiation therapy group is shorter, and thus meaningful comparison between these two treatment groups is not possible. The disease-free 5-year survival after radical prostatectomy alone in pathologic stage-C disease is 50–60% [11,30,33]. These are slightly worse than that of those receiving adjuvant therapy.

In the three intra-institutional studies comparing patients who did or did not receive adjuvant radiation therapy with respect to disease-free survival, no significant difference was appreciated [33,36,40]. The influence of stage migration may have been particularly apparent in the Jacobson series in which the majority of patients who had a lymphadenectomy (precluding radical prostatectomy if positive), and thus probably had a less extensive degree of organ extension, did not receive radiation therapy [36].

The influence of survival of adjuvant radiation therapy in D-1 disease is controversial. While Lange and associates described a 69% 5-year disease-free survival in patients so treated [37], Zincke et al. noted only an 18%

disease-free survival in the group as a whole and 26% of those with only one node. [41].

Smith et al. likewise described disease-free 5-year survival in patients with D-1 disease who had lymphadenectomy without radical prostatectomy and either no adjuvant therapy (29%) or local radiation therapy (17%) at 5 years, thus questioning the importance of the prostatectomy [42].

Recently, Catalona and associates and Steinberg et al. suggested that the 5-year survival of patients with minimal D-1 disease may be greater than previously suggested [29,31]. Again, significant differences between these series with respect to pathological examination and the thoroughness of node dissection, etc. makes a comparison amongst series impossible. Large multicenter prospective randomized studies are currently underway to assess the efficacy of adjuvant external-beam radiation therapy in advanced local prostatic carcinoma.

Prostate specific antigen (PSA) will serve as a meaningful early indicator of the effectiveness of adjuvant therapy. Lange and associates have reported that PSA falls oftentimes to the female serum level following adjuvant external-beam radiation therapy in patients with locally advanced prostate cancer. For example, of 15 men who had persistently detectable PSA follow-up radical prostatectomy, the PSA fell to the female level in 53% following completion of radiation therapy [22].

The durability of the serologic effectiveness of external-beam radiation has, however, recently been questioned by the Stanford group. Link and associates [43] administered external-beam radiation therapy to 26 patients with advanced local disease following radical prostatectomy. Eight were staged D-1 and 18 were Stage C. All had detectable PSA following surgery. Despite the fact that 62% had a decline of PSA to the nondetectable level following radiation therapy, only 2 of 16 patients followed greater than 1 year continued to have nondetectable PSA.

It seems unlikely that subclinical metastatic disease was the source of the persistent PSA in all cases. More likely, it would seem that, despite an effect on persistent carcinoma within the radiation field with a resulting initial decline in PSA, eradication of tumor was not achieved. Obviously, additional studies and longer follow-up in these patients is necessary before definitive conclusions can be made.

Radiation therapy can be given safely in men following radical prostatectomy. Minor complications are common. Diarrhea, skin desquamation, anal pain, and dysuria frequently occur. Usually these are self-limited or can be treated with oral medications. Chronic complications, though rare, may be serious. Ray and associates reported a 31% complication rate in 32 men, including urinary and fecal incontinence [35]. Gibbons and associates reported serious complications occurring in 14% of 22 men, including one requiring colostomy and one requiring a urinary diversion [33].

Lange and associates have described the best results with respect to complications with adjuvant radiation therapy [37]. These authors reported only a 6% complication rating among 71 patients, including only two significant complications. They feel that several factors resulted in their low complication rate, including the performance of a modified pelvic lymphadenectomy with preservation of the lymphatic tissue lateral to the external iliac vessels, limiting the radiation dose to 60 Gy and not starting radiation therapy until the patient is fully recovered from surgery, including the restoration of complete continence.

In conclusion, it would appear that because of the substantial upstaging of men with an apparently clinically localized prostatic carcinoma, there is a need for adjuvant therapy. Improvement in imaging modalities have not offered significant improvement in our ability to properly assess the local stage. Evidence of local disease persistence is likely to improve with the use of more frequent needle biopsy of the region of the vesical urethral anastomosis, perhaps under ultrasound guidance. Clearly, prostate-specific antigen will be pivotal in deciding which patients should be scrutinized for persistent neoplasm.

Despite a considerable body of data on the use of adjuvant radiation therapy, it is difficult to make meaningful comparisons between the studies for a myriad of reasons. Clearly, one must await the results of the ongoing multicenter randomized prospective trials comparing adjuvant radiation therapy and observation following radical prostatectomy in patients with advanced local disease before the true utility of this modality is known.

Acknowledgments

Michael K. Brawer is the recipient as an American Cancer Society Career Development Award. This study was supported in part by a grant from the Veterans Administration.

References

1. Silverberg E, Lubera JA: Cancer Statistics CA 39:3–20.
2. Kabalin JN, Hodge K, McNeal JE, et al.: Identification of residual cancer in the prostate following radiation therapy: Role of transrectal ultrasound guided biopsy and prostate specific antigen. J Urol 142:326–331, 1989.
3. Lange PH, Narayan P: Understaging and undergrading of prostate cancer. Urology 21: 113–118, 1983.
4. Catalona WJ, Stein AJ: Staging errors in clinically localized prostatic cancer. J Urol 127:452–456.
5. Veenema RJ, Gursel EO, Lattimer JK: Radical retropubic prostatectomy for cancer: A 20-year experience. J Urol 117:330–331, 1977.
6. Jewett HJ: The case for radical perineal prostatectomy. J Urol 103:195–199, 1970.
7. Gibbons RP, Correa RJ Jr., Brannen GE, Weissman RM: Total prostatectomy for clinically localized prostatic cancer: Long-term results. J Urol 141:564–566, 1989.
8. Elder JS, Jewett JH, Walsh PC: Radical perineal prostatectomy for clinical stage B_2 carcinoma of the prostate. J Urol 127:704–706, 1982.

9. Spigelman S, McNeal JE, Freiha FS, et al.: Rectal examination in volume determination of carcinoma of the prostate: Clinical and anatomical correlations. J Urol 136:1228–1230, 1986.
10. Carter St. C, Talley D, Egawa S, et al.: Accurate preoperative determination of prostate cancer volume in clinically localized disease. J Urol 141:276A, 1989.
11. Denis L, Appel L, Broos J, et al.: Evaluation of prostatic cancer by transrectal ultrasonography and CT scan. Acta Urol Belg 48:71, 1980.
12. Peeling WB, Griffiths GJ: Imaging of the prostate by ultrasound. J Urol 132:217, 1984.
13. Pontes E, Ohe H, Watanabe H, et al.: Transrectal ultrasonography of the prostate. Cancer 53:1369, 1984.
14. Resnick MI, Willard JW, Boyce WH: Transrectal ultrasonography in the evaluation of patients with prostatic cancer. J Urol 124:226–234, 1980.
15. Lee F: Transrectal ultrasound: Diagnosis and staging of prostatic carcinoma. Urology 33 (Suppl.):5–10, 1989.
16. Stamey TA, McNeal JE, Freiha FS: Morphometric and clinical studies in 68 consecutive radical prostatecomies. J Urol 139:1235, 1988.
17. Lange PH, Moon TD, Narayan P, et al.: Radiation treatment after radical prostatectomy: Patients' tolerance and preliminary results. J Urol 136:45–49, 1986.
18. McNeal JE, Bostwick DG, Kindrachukra, et al.: Patterns of progression in prostatic cancer. Lancet 1:60–63, 1980.
19. Middleton RG, Smith JA Jr., Melzer RM, et al.: Patient survival local recurrence rate following radical prostatectomy following prostatic carcinoma. J Urol 136:422–424, 1986.
20. Villers A, McNeal JE, Redwine EA, Freiha FS, Stamey TA: The role of perineural space invasion in the local spread of prostatic adenocarcinoma. J Urol 142:763–768, 1989.
21. Epstein J: Radical prostatectomy, capsular margins in the margins of resections: The significance of margins designated as negative equivocal and positive. J Urol 143:314A, 1990.
22. Lange PH, Lightner DJ, Medini E, Reddy PK: The effects of radiation therapy after radical prostatectomy in patients with elevated PSA levels J Urol, in press.
23. Lange PH, Ercole CJ, Lightner DJ, Fraley EE, Vessella R: The value of serum prostate specific antigen determinations before and after radical prostatectomy. J Urol 141:873–879, 1989.
24. Hudson MA, Bahnson RB, Catalona WJ: Clinical use of prostate specific antigen in patients with prostate cancer. J Urol, in press.
25. Culp OS: Radical perineal prostatectomy: Its past, present and possible future. J Urol 98:618–626, 1968.
26. Walsh PC, Jewett HJ: Radical surgery for prostatic cancer. Cancer 45:1906–1911.
27. Tomlinson RL, Currie DP, Boyce WH: Radical prostatectomy: Palliation for stage C carcinoma of the prostate. J Urol 117:85–87.
28. Robey EL, Schellhammer PF: Local failure after definitive therapy for prostatic cancer. J Urol 137:613–619.
29. Catalona WJ, Miller DR, Kavoussi LR: Intermediate-term survival results in clinically understaged prostate cancer patients following radical prostatectomy. J Urol 140:540–543.
30. Zincke H, Utz DC, Taylor WF: Bilateral pelvic lymphadenectomy and radical prostatectomy for clinical stage C prostatic cancer: Role of adjuvant treatment for residual cancer and in disease progression. J Urol 135:1199–1205.
31. Steinberg GD, Epstein JI, Piantados S, Walsh PC: Management of stage D1 adenocarcinoma of the prostate: The John Hopkins experience 1974–1987 J Urol 141:310A.
32. Rosenberg SJ, Loening SA, Hawtrey CE, Narayana AS, Culp DA: Radical prostatectomy with adjuvant radioactive gold for prostatic cancer: A preliminary report. J Urol 133: 225–227.
33. Gibbons RP, Cole BS, Richardson RG, Correa RJ Jr., Brannen GE, Mason JT, Taylor WJ, Hafermann MD: Adjuvant radiotherapy following radical prostatectomy: Results and complications. J Urol 135:65–68.

34. Bahnson RR, Garnett JE, Grayhack JT: Adjuvant radiation therapy in stages C and D_1 prostatic adenocarcinoma: Preliminary results. Urology 27:403–406.
35. Ray GR, Bagshaw MA, Freiha F: External beam radiation salvage for residual or recurrent local tumor following radical prostatectomy. J Urol 132:926–930.
36. Jacobson GM, Smith JA Jr., Stewart JR: Postoperative radiation therapy for pathologic stage C prostate cancer. Int J Radiat Oncol Biol Phys 13:1021–1024.
37. Lange PH, Reddy PK, Medini E, Levitt S, Fraley EE: Radiation therapy as adjuvant treatment after radical prostatectomy. NCI Monogr 7:141–149.
38. Pilepich MV, Walz BJ, Baglan RJ: Postoperative irradiation in carcinoma of the prostate. Int J Radiat Oncol Biol Phys 10:1869–1873.
39. Forman JD, Wharam MB, Lee DJ, et al.: Definitive radiotherapy following prostatectomy: Results and complications. Int J Radiat Oncol Biol Phys 12:185–189.
40. Anscher MS, Prosnitz LR: Postoperative radiotherapy for patients with carcinoma of the prostate undergoing radical prostatectomy with positive surgical margins, seminal vesicle involvement and/or penetration through the capsule. J Urol 138:1407–1412.
41. Zincke H, Utz DC, Benson RC Jr., et al.: Bilateral pelvic lymphadenectomy and radical retropubic prostatectomy for stage C adenocarcinoma of prostate. Urology 24:532–539.
42. Smith JA Jr., Haynes TH, Middleton RG: Impact of external irradiation on local symptoms and survival free of disease in patients with pelvic lymph node metastasis from adenocarcinoma of the prostate. J Urol 131:705–707.
43. Link P, Freiha FS, Stamey TA: Adjuvant radiation therapy in patients with detectable prostatic specific antigen following radical prostatectomy. J Urol, in press.

5. Nuclear DNA ploidy and prostate cancer

Leslie M. Rainwater and Horst Zincke

Prostate cancer is now the most common cancer in men in the United States [1]. Although 103,000 new cases were expected in 1989, less than one third were projected to die of their disease. The vast majority of prostate cancer remains clinically undetectable for the patient's entire life. This discrepancy in the biologic behavior of prostate cancer remains a mystery. However, attempting to determine which tumors will remain indolent and which will follow an aggressive course is the work of much investigation.

Prior to recent developments, clinicians relied on histologic grading to determine the biologic behavior of tumors [2–6]. Grading appears to be a good indicator of biologic behavior in both extremes, i.e., well-differentiated tumors and poorly differentiated tumors. However, the majority of tumors remain in the moderately differentiated category, and histologic grading remains a subjective classification and can vary because of day-to-day differences in interpretation.

Clinical and pathologic staging appears to play a role in determining biologic behavior, but clinical staging may correlate with pathologic staging in only 50% of cases [7,8]. Within a given pathologic stage, there is variability in the biologic behavior of a given tumor. Therefore, investigations have begun focusing on the quantitative analysis of tumor nuclear DNA ploidy patterns as an objective way to determine the biologic behavior of prostate adenocarcinoma.

In 1966, Tavares et al. [9] first reported on the correlation between tumor DNA ploidy and prostate cancer by using static cytomorphometry. These investigators found 7 of 26 patients (27%) with DNA diploid or DNA tetraploid (2C/4C) tumors died, with a mean survival of 7.4 years, compared to 7 of 9 patients (78%) having DNA aneuploid (3C/6C) tumors who died with a mean survival of 4.1 years. Furthermore, 92% of tumors with a DNA diploid or DNA tetraploid pattern responded to estrogen therapy, as opposed to 89% of tumors with a DNA aneuploid pattern that were resistant to estrogen therapy. In a follow-up article in 1973 with 76 patients, these same findings were reiterated [10]. However, static cytomorphometry is a time-consuming process that is based on the analysis of a limited number of cells, i.e., 30–300 cells. Thus, flow cytometric analysis of tumor nuclear

Lepor, H. and Lawson R.K., (eds.), Therapy for Genitourinary Cancer.
Kluwer Academic Publishers. ISBN 0-7923-1412-3.

DNA was developed; it allows for rapid quantification of 10,000–100,000 cells in a matter of minutes but does require a single-cell suspension of the tumor specimen.

In 1977, Bichel et al. [11] described the use of flow cytometric analysis of transrectal fine-needle prostate aspirates to characterize prostate adenocarcinoma. Their investigations, confirmed by others [12–14], demonstrated the presence of abnormal DNA ploidy patterns, DNA tetraploid and DNA aneuploid, and correlated these patterns with increasing histologic anaplasia of the prostate tumors studied. Poorly differentiated tumors had almost exclusively abnormal DNA ploidy patterns. Moderately differentiated tumors had an admixture of patterns: Some were DNA diploid, whereas others were DNA aneuploid or DNA tetraploid. Pontes et al. [8] performed flow cytometric analysis on 33 radical prostatectomy specimens. Nuclear DNA ploidy analysis combined with Gleason's score improved the predictive value of the histologic grading in high-stage lesions. Although these aforementioned studies correlated increasing histologic grading with an increasing incidence of DNA aneuploidy, little correlation could be made between DNA ploidy and patient prognosis or the time to progression because of the short-term follow-up. Indeed, follow-up of 10–15 years seems to be required for determining the positive predictive value of nuclear DNA ploidy analysis.

In 1983 Hedley and associates [15] first described a method for extracting a single-cell nucleus from formalin-fixed, paraffin-embedded archival pathologic material for analysis by flow cytometry. The modified Hedley method used at our institution has been described [16]: one to two 50-μm sections are cut on a standard microtome from the paraffin-embedded tissue block. These sections are placed in a 10-ml glass culture tube and then dewaxed in two changes of Histoclear (National Diagnostic, Somerville, NJ), 3 ml for 10 minutes at room temperature. The tissue specimens are rehydrated in a sequence of ethanol/water solutions (3 ml) of 100%, 90%, and 70% ethanol for 5 minutes at room temperature. The dewaxed tissue specimens are washed twice in distilled water and resuspended in 0.5% pepsin (1 ml) in normal saline adjusted to pH 1.5. These specimens are incubated at 37°C for 90 minutes in a water bath with intermittent mixing (vortex). This is followed by low-speed centrifugation to pellet the nuclei, and the pepsin-containing supernatant is removed. Thereby, the nuclei are freed from the paraffin blocks and are ready to be stained for analysis in the flow cytometer system. Our institution uses the fluorescent dye propidium iodide, which binds the DNA and gives a quantitative fluorescent measurement of nuclear DNA content, as described by Vindeløv et al. [17]. Other staining techniques have been described that use propidium iodide [18], DAPI [19] (4′,6-diamidino-2-phenylindole dihydrochloride), ethridium bromide [20], and mithramycin [21]. The methodology described by Hedley and associates [15] allowed the analysis of various genitourinary tumors to determine the correlation between nuclear DNA ploidy with tumor progression, tumor response to chemotherapeutic agents, and patient prognosis [22–26].

Since 1986 several investigators have reported on the use of paraffin-embedded archival material to perform flow cytometry. Fordham et al. [27] reported on 72 patients who had undergone prostatectomy for adenocarcinoma and had up to a 12-year follow-up. The majority (73%) had some form of hormonal manipulation as the primary treatment and 22% had radiotherapy. Both the Gleason score and DNA ploidy predicted patient survival. However, combining the Gleason score with DNA ploidy was highly predictive of patient prognosis. One hundred percent of patients died with a DNA aneuploid pattern and a Gleason score of 7–10 at 3 years (mean survival 22.4 months), whereas only 17% of patients died with a DNA diploid pattern and a Gleason score of 2–6 at 3 years (mean survival 104.5 months). Patients with a high Gleason score of 7–10 and a DNA diploid pattern, or a low Gleason score of 2–6 and a DNA aneuploid pattern, had intermediate survival of 55.2 months and 68.0 months, respectively.

McIntire et al. [28] reported on the prognostic value of DNA ploidy for incidental carcinoma (stage A1 and A2) of the prostate. Of the patients with stage A2 and a DNA aneuploid pattern, 67% progressed, compared to 0% of patients with stage A1 and a DNA diploid pattern. The one patient with a stage A1 tumor and DNA aneuploid progressed, whereas only 15% of patients with a stage A2 and a DNA diploid pattern progressed. DNA ploidy pattern correlated significantly with progression in stage A1 and stage A2 tumors (Table 1).

Blute and associates [29] performed DNA flow cytometric analysis on tumors of 38 patients who had undergone a radical retropubic prostatectomy with organ-confined disease (pathologic stage A and stage B) who suffered progression and 38 age-matched controls. Various prognostic variables were examined, and only DNA tumor ploidy predicted progression significantly (Table 2). Ninety-two percent of tumors in the control group were DNA

Table 1. Tumor progression shown by DNA ploidy pattern

		Progression[a]							
		Diploid		Tetraploid		Aneuploid		Tetraploid + Aneuploid (Abnormal)	
Pathologic Stage	No. Patients	No.	%	No.	%	No.	%	No.	%
A1 [28]	11	10	0	—		—		1	100
A2 [28]	22	13	15	—		—		9	67
B [29]	261	177	15	74	22	10	100	84	31
C [30]	146	67	19	68	50	11	64	79	52
D1 [31]	91	38	15	41	74	12	80	53	75

[a] Local or systemic progression.

Table 2. Pathologic variables and DNA tumor ploidy determined by flow cytometry for 76 patients who underwent bilateral pelvic lymph-node dissection and radical retropubic prostatectomy without adjuvant treatment for clinically and pathologically confined adenocarcinoma of the prostate

	Group 1		Group 2		
	No.	%	No.	%	p Value
Mayo grade					
1–2	23	61	28	74	0.30
3–4	15	39	10	26	
Gleason score					
3–5	13	34	15	39	0.36
6–9	25	66	23	61	
Tumor volume, cm^3					
<3	30	79	28	74	0.99
3–10	7	18	9	24	
>10	1	3	1	3	
Multifocal					
No	28	74	27	71	0.99
Yes	10	26	11	29	
Capsular invasion					
Yes	25	66	17	45	0.48
No	13	34	21	55	
DNA tumor ploidy					
Diploid	14	37	35	92	0.0004
Tetraploid	13 } 24	63	3 } 3[a]	8	
Aneuploid	11		0		

Group 1, 38 patients who experienced progression (local/systemic).
Group 2, 38 age-matched controls who did not experience progression.
[a] Follow-up for these patients is 14, 12, and 7 years. (From Blute et al. [29]. By permission of Williams and Wilkins.)

diploid, and no tumors exhibited a DNA aneuploid pattern. Of the 38 patients who progressed, 24 tumors had abnormal DNA ploidy patterns (DNA tetraploid and DNA aneuploid), 63% of which failed systemically and 37% failed locally. In the eight patients who progressed with DNA diploid tumors, 57% failed locally and 43% failed systemically. In a follow-up study, Montgomery and associates [32] reported on 261 patients who had undergone radical retropubic prostatectomy for pathologic stage B prostate adenocarcinoma. The ploidy distribution was as follows: 177 (68%) were DNA diploid; 74 (28%) were DNA tetraploid; and 10 (4%) were DNA aneuploid. Within the study group, 53 patients' tumors had progressed: 22 locally, 23 systemically, and 8 both, with a mean follow-up of 9.4 years. Overall, 31% of nondiploid tumors progressed (22% DNA tetraploid and 100% DNA aneuploid), compared to 15% of DNA diploid tumors. DNA ploidy analysis had marked prognostic significance for patients with pathologic stage B tumors (Table 1).

Lee et al. [30] reported on 80 deparaffinized radical prostatectomy specimens, comparing DNA ploidy as a predictor of disease progression to Gleason score and seminal vesicle involvement. Their study showed DNA ploidy correlated with the stage of the tumor and predicted tumor progression. Patients with tumors with a DNA diploid pattern had an 85% disease-free survival at 5 years compared to only 9% disease-free survival for patients with tumors with a DNA aneuploid pattern at 5 years. Patients with seminal vesicle involvement and DNA diploid tumors had a 73% nonprogression compared to only an 8% nonprogression rate with DNA aneuploid tumors. Further, all 18 patients without seminal vesicle involvement and a DNA diploid pattern are free of disease at 5-year follow-up. There was a 29% recurrence rate in intermediate-grade tumors (Gleason 5–7), but only a 5% recurrence rate in intermediate-grade DNA diploid tumors. In conclusion, these authors found a DNA aneuploid stem line to correlate statistically with a greater likelihood of seminal vesicle invasion and subsequent development of recurrent disease.

Nativ and associates [33] examined 146 patients' tumors with pathologic stage C (pT3, N0, M0) who underwent radical prostatectomy for adenocarcinoma. The DNA ploidy distribution was as follows: 67 (46%) had a DNA diploid pattern; 68 (47%) had a DNA tetraploid pattern; and 11 (7%) had a DNA aneuploid pattern. An abnormal ploidy pattern (DNA tetraploid and DNA aneuploid) was associated more frequently with histologic high-grade tumors. The median interval to progression for DNA tetraploid and DNA aneuploid tumors was 7.8 and 3.5 years, respectively. At 10-year follow-up, only 10% of patients with DNA diploid tumors died of disease, compared to 28% and 36% of DNA tetraploid and DNA aneuploid tumors, respectively, which was significant. The combination of histologic tumor grade and nuclear DNA ploidy demonstrated an even stronger prognostic association. For low-grade DNA diploid tumors, progression-free survival was 92% at 10 years, compared to only 57% progression-free survival for low-grade DNA nondiploid tumors. For this group of patients with pathologic stage C disease, nuclear DNA ploidy pattern proved to be an independent prognostic indicator of disease progression (Table 1).

Stephenson et al. [31] performed flow cytometric analysis on paraffin-embedded tumor specimens from 82 patients with pathologic stage D1 who had been treated with pelvic lymph-node dissection and iodine-125 seed implants. Thirty-three tumors were DNA diploid and 49 tumors were DNA aneuploid. The median survival was significantly longer for patients with DNA diploid vs. DNA aneuploid tumors: 8.8 vs. 5.0 years, respectively. Grade, as a predictor of survival, did not reach statistical significance. Among the moderately differentiated tumors, the median survival for patients with DNA diploid vs. DNA aneuploid tumors was 9.1 vs. 5.8 years, respectively. These authors found DNA ploidy patterns to be a strong predictor of survival for stage D1 prostate adenocarcinoma.

Winkler and associates [34] examined paraffin-embedded tumor specimens from 91 patients who had undergone radical retropubic prostatectomy for pathologic stage D1 adenocarcinoma. The DNA ploidy patterns were as follows: 38 (42%) had a DNA diploid pattern, 41 (45%) had a DNA tetraploid pattern, and 12 (13%) had a DNA aneuploid pattern. Only 15% of DNA diploid tumors progressed locally or systemically, compared to 75% of tumors with an abnormal DNA ploidy pattern. None of the patients with a DNA diploid pattern died of prostate cancer, whereas 43% of patients with DNA tetraploid tumors and 44% of patients with DNA aneuploid tumors died of prostate cancer. Only 12% of patients with low-grade tumors (Gleason score 2–5) and a DNA diploid pattern progressed, whereas 67% with a DNA tetraploid pattern and 100% with a DNA aneuploid pattern progressed. Only 18% of patients with high-grade tumors (Gleason score 6–10) and a DNA diploid pattern progressed, whereas 77% with a DNA tetraploid pattern and 75% with a DNA aneuploid pattern progressed. Therefore, nuclear DNA ploidy analysis represents an objective prognostic indicator for patients with stage D1 prostate cancer, which proved to be highly significant (Table 1).

Several investigators have found DNA ploidy analysis to be a means of monitoring the effects of treatment responses to luteinizing hormone-releasing factor (LHRH) analogues and hormonal manipulation [12,35–39]. A change of DNA ploidy from DNA aneuploid to DNA diploid correlated with a favorable response [12,35]. Furthermore, DNA diploid tumors appear to respond more favorably to LHRH analogues or hormonal manipulation than do tumors with an abnormal DNA ploidy pattern [36,37]. These findings were confirmed in a group of 176 patients with pathologic stage D1 disease who had undergone radical prostatectomy with or without hormonal treatment and were followed for up to 21 years (median 5.4 years) [38,39]. Sixty-nine patients' tumors (39%) had a DNA diploid pattern, whereas the remaining 107 patients' tumors (61%) had a nondiploid DNA ploidy pattern. None of the 50 patients with a DNA diploid tumor and immediate adjuvant hormonal treatment progressed; however, 10 of 19 patients with no adjuvant treatment progressed ($p < 0.00001$) (Figure 1). Furthermore, 3 of 10 patients who progressed with DNA diploid tumors died of their disease at an average of 19 months (range, 2–56 months), despite prompt hormonal therapy initiated at the first signs of clinical progression ($p < 0.019$) (Figure 2). DNA nondiploid tumors were also associated with better disease outcome with regard to progression when treated with immediate adjuvant hormonal therapy (Figure 1), but this was not of statistical significance when cause-specific survival was analyzed (Figure 2) [39].

Correlations between DNA ploidy pattern and increased prostate-specific antigen (PSA) levels were suggested previously [40]; however, when a large number of patients was analyzed ($n = 146$), no significant difference could be found between the various DNA ploidy patterns and an increased PSA level (>4.0 ml). Eighty-one percent of patients with a DNA diploid pattern,

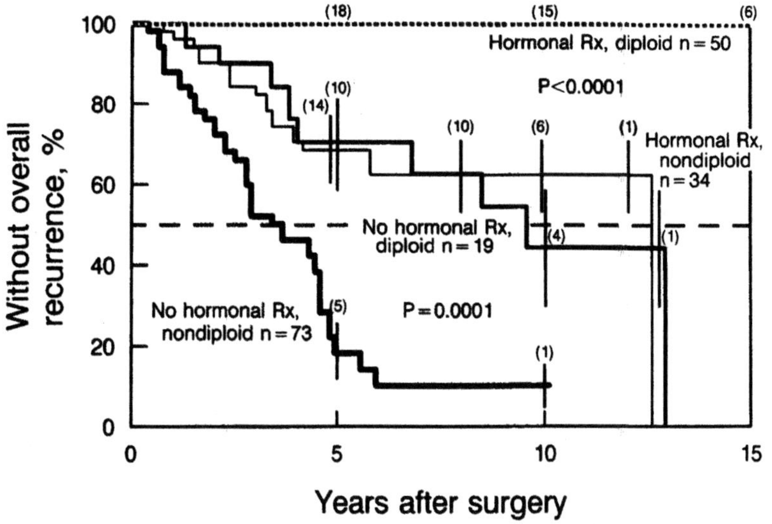

Figure 1. Kaplan-Meier curves of overall survival without recurrence in 176 patients with stage D1 prostate cancer who underwent radical prostatectomy according to adjuvant treatment and the tumor nuclear-DNA ploidy pattern. The numbers in parentheses represent patients under observation at that time.

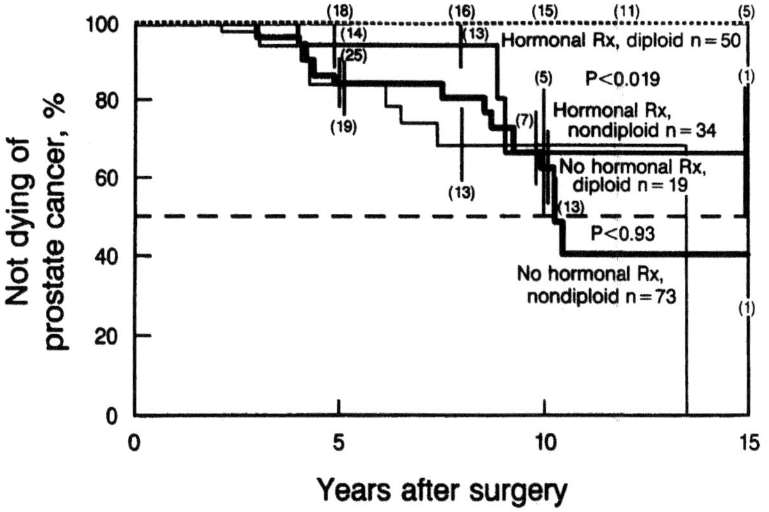

Figure 2. Kaplan-Meier curves of cause-specific survival in 176 patients with stage D1 prostate cancer who underwent radical prostatectomy according to adjuvant treatment and the tumor nuclear-DNA ploidy pattern. The numbers in parentheses represent patients under observation at that time. (From Zincke [39]. By permission of W.B. Saunders Company.)

84% with a DNA tetraploid pattern, and 86% with a DNA aneuploid pattern had an increased PSA level preoperatively (L.M. Rainwater, H. Zincke, unpublished data). Not only is there a correlation between tumor size and an increased PSA level, but there is also a conspicuous relationship between increasing tumor size or age, or both, and DNA ploidy.

In study after study from various institutions around the world, nuclear DNA ploidy analysis has proved to be an independent prognostic variable. Although nuclear DNA ploidy cannot be used to diagnose cancer [13,41,42], knowledge that a tumor has a DNA diploid stem line of cells does correlate with a more indolent nature of the primary tumor and decreased potential for future local or systemic recurrences. In contrast, an abnormal DNA ploidy pattern, in particular a DNA aneuploid stem line of cells, portends a more virulent tumor, for which one would anticipate a local or systemic recurrence that will respond poorly to LHRH analogues or hormonal therapy.

Tumor heterogeneity of prostate cancer has been noted previously in histologic tumor specimens. However, histologically similar tumor specimens have now been found with the use of flow cytometry to have nuclear DNA ploidy heterogeneity, further substantiating the variability in biologic behavior [13,19]. In prostate cancer, which has a diverse biologic behavior, the addition of an objective independent prognostic variable, nuclear DNA ploidy analysis, opens the possibilities for future studies comparing various treatment modalities. In the future, additional parameters may also be obtained for evaluating prostatic cancer cells, including relative cell size, protein content, 5α-reductase activity, or various cytoplasmic constituents by using multiple-laser, flow cytometric systems, which will allow for further classification of the heterogeneous biologic behavior of prostate tumor specimens [43–46].

Now more than ever it is imperative for studies relating to radiotherapy, radical surgery, use of LHRH analogues, hormonal therapy, and chemotherapy alone or as an adjuvant to definitive local therapy to include nuclear DNA ploidy for future comparative analyses. For instance, some of the recently reported data, in particular those with the surgical treatment of stage D1 and adjuvant hormonal treatment [39], can only be intelligently interpreted with the help of tumor nuclear DNA ploidy analysis. Hence, any prospective study concerning the treatment of prostate cancer should include DNA ploidy analysis as a most important disease variable.

With the use of PSA in combination with ultrasonographically guided biopsies of the prostate and blind random-sampling biopsies, previously undetectable tumors are now being found routinely. However, are we now overtreating these clinically undetectable tumors that would have remained silent and indolent had not sophisticated diagnostic techniques been developed? Future studies that include nuclear DNA ploidy analysis of the tumor specimens may indicate which tumor requires aggressive radical surgery, which will respond to hormonal or chemotherapeutic agents, and which can be followed by expectant observation alone.

References

1. Silverberg E, Lubera JA: Cancer Statistics. CA 39:3–20, 1989.
2. Utz DC, Farrow GM: Pathologic differentiation and prognosis of prostatic carcinoma. JAMA 209:1701–1703, 1969.
3. Mostofi FK: Problems of grading carcinoma of prostate. Semin Oncol 3:161–169, 1976.
4. Gaeta JF, Asirwatham JE, Miller G, Murphy GP: Histologic grading of primary prostatic cancer: A new approach to an old problem. J Urol 123:689–693, 1980.
5. Brawn PN, Ayala AG, von Eschenbach AC, Hussey DH, Johnson DE: Histologic grading study of prostate adenocarcinoma: The development of a new system and comparison with other methods — a preliminary study. Cancer 49:525–532, 1982.
6. Gleason DF, The Veterans Administration Cooperative Urological Research Group: Histologic grading and clinical staging of prostatic carcinoma. In: *Urologic Pathology: The Prostate*. Tannenbaum M (ed). Lea and Febiger, Philadelphia, 1977, pp. 171–197.
7. Zincke H: Bilateral pelvic lymphadenectomy and radical retropubic prostatectomy for stage C or D1 adenocarcinoma of the prostate: Possible beneficial effect of adjuvant treatment. Natl Cancer Inst Monogr 7:109–115, 1988.
8. Pontes JE, Wajsman Z, Huben RP, Wolf RM, Englander LS: Prognostic factors in localized prostatic carcinoma. J Urol 134:1137–1139, 1985.
9. Tavares AS, Costa J, de Carvalho A, Reis M: Tumour ploidy and prognosis in carcinomas of the bladder and prostate. Br J Cancer 20:438–441, 1966.
10. Tavares AS, Costa J, Costa Maia J: Correlation between ploidy and prognosis in prostatic carcinoma. J Urol 109:676–679, 1973.
11. Bichel P, Frederiksen P, Kjaer T, Thommesen P, Vindeløv LL: Flow microfluorometry and transrectal fine-needle biopsy in the classification of human prostatic carcinoma. Cancer 40:1206–1211, 1977.
12. Zetterberg A, Esposti PL: Prognostic significance of nuclear DNA levels in prostatic carcinoma. Scand J Urol Nephrol 55:53–58, 1980.
13. Rönström L, Tribukait B, Esposti PL: DNA pattern and cytological findings in fine-needle aspirates of untreated prostatic tumors: A flow-cytofluorometric study. Prostate 2:79–88, 1981.
14. Roters M, Laemmel A, Kastendieck H, Becker H: DNA distribution pattern of prostatic lesions measured by flow cytometry. Acta Pathol Microbiol Scand [A] (Suppl.) 274: 431–435, 1981.
15. Hedley DW, Friedlander ML, Taylor IW, Rugg CA, Musgrove EA: Method for analysis of cellular DNA content of paraffin-embedded pathological material using flow cytometry. J Histochem Cytochem 31:1333–1335, 1983.
16. Rainwater LM, Lieber MM: New uses for old nuclei: DNA ploidy pattern and prognosis for patients with genitourinary neoplasms. In: *Urology Annual*, Vol. 2. Rous SN (ed). Appleton and Lange, Norwalk, CT, 1988, pp. 27–46.
17. Vindeløv LL, Christensen IJ, Nissen NI: A detergent-trypsin method for the preparation of nuclei for flow cytometric DNA analysis. Cytometry 3:323–327, 1983.
18. Lee SE, Currin SM, Paulson DF, Walther PJ: Flow cytometric determination of ploidy in prostatic adenocarcinoma: A comparison with seminal vesicle involvement and histopathological grading as a predictor of clinical recurrence. J Urol 140:769–774, 1988.
19. Lundberg S, Carstensen J, Rundquist I: DNA flow cytometry and histopathological grading of paraffin-embedded prostate biopsy specimens in a survival study. Cancer Res 47: 1973–1977, 1987.
20. Le Pecq J-B, Paoletti C: A new fluorometric method for RNA and DNA determination. Anal Biochem 17:100–107, 1966.
21. Crissman HA, Tobey RA: Cell-cycle analysis in 20 minutes. Science 184:1297–1298, 1974.
22. Rainwater LM, Hosaka Y, Farrow GM, Lieber MM: Well differentiated clear cell renal carcinoma: Significance of nuclear deoxyribonucleic acid patterns studied by flow cytometry. J Urol 137:15–20, 1987.

23. Rainwater LM, Hosaka Y, Farrow GM, Kramer SA, Kelalis PP, Lieber MM: Wilms tumors: Relationship of nuclear deoxyribonucleic acid ploidy to patient survival. J Urol 138:974–977, 1987.
24. Hosaka Y, Rainwater LM, Grant CS, Farrow GM, van Heerden JA, Lieber MM: Pheochromocytoma: Nuclear deoxyribonucleic acid patterns studied by flow cytometry. Surgery 100:1003–1008, 1986.
25. Hosaka Y, Rainwater LM, Grant CS, Young WF Jr., Farrow GM, van Heerden JA, Lieber MM: Adrenocortical carcinoma: Nuclear deoxyribonucleic acid ploidy studied by flow cytometry. Surgery 102:1027–1033, 1987.
26. Boyle ET Jr., Reiman HM, Kramer SA, Kelalis PP, Rainwater LM, Lieber MM: Embryonal rhabdomyosarcoma of bladder and prostate: Nuclear DNA patterns studied by flow cytometry. J Urol 140:1119–1121, 1988.
27. Fordham MVP, Burdge AH, Matthews J, Williams G, Cooke T: Prostatic carcinoma cell DNA content measured by flow cytometry and its relation to clinical outcome. Br J Surg 73:400–403, 1986.
28. McIntire TL, Murphy WM, Coon JS, Chandler RW, Schwartz D, Conway S, Weinstein RS: The prognostic value of DNA ploidy combined with histologic substaging for incidental carcinoma of the prostate gland. Am J Clin Pathol 89:370–373, 1988.
29. Blute ML, Nativ O, Zincke H, Farrow GM, Therneau T, Lieber MM: Pattern of failure after radical retropubic prostatectomy for clinically and pathologically localized adenocarcinoma of the prostate: Influence of tumor deoxyribonucleic acid ploidy. J Urol 142: 1262–1265, 1989.
30. Lee SE, Currin SM, Paulson DF, Walther PJ: Flow cytometric determination of ploidy in prostatic adenocarcinoma: A comparison with seminal vesicle involvement and histopathological grading as a predictor of clinical recurrence. J Urol 140:769–774, 1988.
31. Stephenson RA, James BC, Gay H, Fair WR, Whitmore WF Jr., Melamed MR: Flow cytometry of prostate cancer: Relationship of DNA content to survival. Cancer Res 47:2504–2509, 1987.
32. Montgomery BT, Nativ O, Blute ML, Farrow GM, Myers RP, Zincke H, Therneau TM, Lieber MM: Stage B prostatic adenocarcinoma: Flow cytometric nuclear DNA ploidy analysis. Arch Surg 125:327–331, 1990.
33. Nativ O, Winkler HZ, Raz Y, Therneau TM, Farrow GM, Myers RP, Zincke H, Lieber MM: Stage C prostatic adenocarcinoma: Flow cytometric nuclear DNA ploidy analysis. Mayo Clin Proc 64:911–919, 1989.
34. Winkler HZ, Rainwater LM, Myers RP, Farrow GM, Therneau TM, Zincke H, Lieber MM: Stage D1 prostatic adenocarcinoma: Significance of nuclear DNA ploidy patterns studied by flow cytometry. Mayo Clin Proc 63:103–112, 1988.
35. Koss LG, Woyke S, Schreiber K, Kohlberg W, Freed SZ: Thin-needle aspiration biopsy of the prostate. Urol Clin North Am 11(2):237–251, 1984.
36. Kjaer TB, Thommesen P, Frederiksen P, Bichel P: DNA content in cells aspirated from carcinoma of the prostate treated with oestrogenic compounds. Urol Res 7:249–251, 1979.
37. Borgmann V, Al-Abadi H, Nagel R: Treatment of locally advanced prostatic carcinoma with LHRH analogues: Cytological, DNA-cytophotometrical, and clinical results. Am J Clin Oncol 11 (Suppl. 1):S19–S28, 1988.
38. Zincke H: Extended experience with surgical treatment of stage D1 adenocarcinoma of prostate: Significant influences of immediate adjuvant hormonal treatment (orchiectomy) on outcome. Urology 33 (Suppl. 5):27–36, 1989.
39. Zincke, H: Combined surgery and immediate adjuvant hormonal treatment for stage D1 adenocarcinoma of the prostate: Mayo Clinic experience. Semin Urol 8:175–183, 1990.
40. Nativ O, Myers RP, Farrow GM, Therneau TM, Zincke H, Lieber MM: Nuclear deoxyribonucleic acid ploidy and serum prostate specific antigen in operable prostatic adenocarcinoma. J Urol 144:303–306, 1990.
41. Benson, MC: Application of flow cytometry and automated image analysis to the study of prostate cancer. Natl Cancer Inst Monogr 7:25–29, 1988.

42. Lieber MM: Editorial comment. J Urol 142:762, 1989.
43. Benson MC: The application of flow cytometry to the study of prostate cancer. Prog Clin Biol Res 239:765–778, 1987.
44. Pollack A, Moulis H, Block NL, Irvin GL, III: Quantitation of cell kinetic responses using simultaneous flow cytometric measurements of DNA and nuclear protein. Cytometry 5:473–481, 1984.
45. Schultz RE, Varello MA, Tsou KC, Wein AJ, Murphy JJ: Simultaneous flow cytometric deoxyribonucleic acid and acid phosphatase analysis of benign and malignant lesions of the prostate. J Urol 134:1133–1136, 1985.
46. Habib FK, Bissas A, Neill WA, Busuttil A, Chisholm GD: Flow cytometric analysis of cellular DNA in human prostate cancer: Relationship to 5 α-reductase activity of the tissue. Urol Res 17:239–243, 1989.

6. Brachytherapy of localized penile carcinoma

R.W. Byhardt and J.F. Wilson

Radiation therapy, administered either by external beam or interstitial implantation (brachytherapy), plays an important role in the management of penile squamous carcinoma. Selection of appropriate cases for radiation treatment using brachytherapy techniques depends on an understanding of the epidemiology, pathobiology, and staging of the disease.

Epidemiology and pathobiology of penile cancer

Squamous cell carcinoma of the penis accounts for only 1% of all malignancies in males in the United States [3], although its incidence may approach 20% in other cultures where retained foreskin and resultant poor penile hygiene play an etiologic role [10,27]. Age at presentation may range from the fourth to ninth decades, with most appearing in the mid-60s [28]. The majority of lesions occur in the glans, but are often present as advanced local disease, often with accompanying nodal involvement, precluding function preserving local therapy of the primary lesion. This is partly due to delay in seeking medical advice because of ignorance, embarassment, neglect, or fear of loss of the organ [12,15,25,34]. Less well-differentiated, more aggressive lesions tend to occur in younger men [9]. Primary treatment is often surgical, but smaller, limited lesions offer a possibility of organ preservation with brachytherapy.

Staging

Two clinical staging systems are in use (Table 1), namely, that of Jackson, based on depth of infiltration [16], and the TNM classification, based on size [11]. The TNM system is preferred for identifying cases suitable for brachytherapy, since it takes better account of primary tumor size, which has demonstrated prognostic value [7] and bears on the selection of brachytherapy as a feasible form of therapy for the primary lesion [2]. If nodal disease is at high risk or present, in association with a T1, T2, or limited

Lepor, H. and Lawson R.K., (eds.), Therapy for Genitourinary Cancer.
Kluwer Academic Publishers. ISBN 0-7923-1412-3.

Table 1. The Jackson [15] and TNM/UICC (10) staging systems

	TNM (UICC)	Jackson
Stage I	T1-2, N0, M0	Limited to glans/prepuce; no nodes or metastases
Stage II	T1-2, N0, M0	Extends to shaft/corpora; no nodes or metastases
Stage III	T1-3, N1-2, M0	Confined to glans/shaft; operable nodes; no mets
Stage IV	T1-4, N0-4, M0-1	Beyond glans/shaft; inoperable nodes and/or distant metastases

T1 = 2 cm or less; T2 = 2 to 5 cm, minimal infiltration; T3 = >5 cm or deep infiltration to urethra; T4 = infiltration of neighboring structures.

T3 primary lesion suitable for implantation, brachytherapy may still be provided, along with surgical or external beam irradiation of the nodal disease if organ preservation is a treatment goal.

Factors influencing choice of therapy

The patient's age and medical fitness also influence the choice of treatment. Although some authors advocate partial penectomy even for small, localized lesions [27,36], most would favor organ-sparing therapy where possible. Functional disability and psychological trauma associated with penile amputation (even partial) probably exceeds that associated with mastectomy, approaching that of abdomino-perineal resection. There are reports of suicide after penectomy [10]. Thus, it is advantageous to attempt local control with preservation of function, both urinary and sexual.

Radiation therapy is felt by many to be the treatment of choice for early disease [4,5,8,9,13,14,19,22,23,26,29–33,35], with occasional success in advanced lesions, although some others remain more circumspect in advocating radiation therapy [7,17,38]. In the event of local failure following irradiation, salvage surgery, usually partial penectomy, often achieves tumor control.

Radiation therapy for penile cancer

Radium molds and external beam

Radiotherapeutic approaches to penile cancer have evolved considerably over the past several decades, with studies in the 1960s and 1970s employing external superficial x-ray therapy or radium molds, with these modalities providing local control rates ranging from 32% to 65% [18,21,24]. More recent data describe local control rates of 67–92%, with external radiation therapy using various types of treatment aids and positioning devices [9,

20,32,33]. These treatment aids, fabricated of tissue-equivalent material (plastic or wax), ensure dose uniformity and overcome skin-sparing effects of high-energy x-rays, which would otherwise result in an underdosage of the superficial component of penile cancers. These all have the relative disadvantages of skin and mucosal (urethral) reactions over a generally greater area of the penis and a more prolonged treatment course (50–60 Gy in 5–6 weeks) than with brachytherapy. The acute effects do clear within several weeks of completion, but there is a risk of late skin telangiectasia or fibrosis of the corpora.

Brachytherapy

Brachytherapy implies the technique of irradiating tumors from a short distance to minimize exposure of the normal tissues surrounding the tumor. This is accomplished by the placement, usually temporary, of radioactive sources directly into and/or around the tumor. Implantation of radioactive sources directly into the lesion has the advantage of limiting the irradiated volume to that of the tumor volume, plus a limited "margin" of uninvolved tissue, as well as a shorter total treatment time (usually 3–4 days) compared to fractionated external beam irradiation, which extends over several weeks. There is also a potential radiobiologic advantage, in terms of a favorable differential in tumor cell killing vs. normal tissue effects, to the delivery of the radiation at a continuous low dose rate, in contrast to the fractionated high doses used with external beam therapy (teletherapy or irradiation from a long distance). Acute skin and mucosal reactions to brachytherapy are also more confined in area, and the risk of extensive late radiation changes is decreased compared to teletherapy, although there is still a risk of localized late effects.

Brachytherapy with radium-226 needles [9] has been supplanted by the use of iridium-192 made into wires or seed trains [4,23,31]. Much of this development has been pioneered by several French brachytherapy centers, with excellent results [2,23,31]. The iridium-192 type sources have the advantages of greater miniaturization and flexibility than radium-226. This allows use of an "afterloading" technique, in which inert guide needles or catheters are first implanted into the tumor area until the correct geometry is achieved; only then are the radioactive sources "afterloaded" into the guides, limiting radiation exposure to personnel. Various computerized systems are used to precisely calculate the distribution of radiation dose (dosimetry) from such implantations.

Brachytherapy clinical series

Both Mazeron [23] and Daly [4], in recent series, have advocated iridium-192 interstitial implant over external techniques based on improved local control, especially for invasive T3 lesions (Table 2). Mazeron noted that

Table 2. Summary of clinical results with iridium 192 wire brachytherapy in early penile carcinoma

Author	Local Control with Retained Penis	Surgical Salvage Tumor	Surgery for Necrosis	Ultimate Tumor Control	Urethral Stenosis
Mazeron [22]	34/45	10/11[a]	3/3	44/45	8/34[b]
Daly [3]	19/22	1/1	2/2	22/22	9/21[b]
Adams [1]	4/8	1/1	1/1	6/8	0/4

[a] One patient refused surgery.
[b] Usually treated with dilatation.

improvement in local control was limited to distal lesions less than 4 cm in diameter, with either no or moderate infiltration of the corpora. Overall, Daly achieved local control with organ preservation in 85% of T1, T2, and T3 lesions. Mazeron observed local control with organ preservation in 74% (80% if the lesion was less than 4 cm and superficially invasive). In both series, ultimate local control after salvage surgery for recurrences was 100%.

The influence of tumor size on local control and overall survival has been noted in other studies as well, most recently by Fraley [7]. This underscores a pitfall of using the Jackson staging system [16], which can include three T stages under Stage I (T1, T2, and T3 lesions less than 5 cm with infiltration to the urethra), thus, somewhat obscuring the effect of tumor size on prognosis (Table 1). As tumor size increases, in addition to an increasing risk of local recurrence, the implanted volume must also increase, with a consequent increase in the risk of radionecrosis or stricture. Brachytherapy is not usually advised for lesions over 4 cm in diameter.

Overall, Mazeron noted urethral stenosis in 8/34 (23%) of patients; 3/8 required surgical correction. Daly observed stenosis in 9/21 (43%) at 10–18 months postimplant, most of which were successfully treated with dilatation. In 5–10% of patients, localized necrosis at the tumor site may simulate tumor recurrence and may require penile amputation (Table 2). Both studies demonstrated that sexual function was usually normal following iridium-192 implant. The potential risk of radiation-induced secondary penile cancers following implant is negligible according to Grabstaldt [8].

In a series of 26 patients with penile cancer seen at the Medical College of Wisconsin since 1974 by the authors, eight (1 T1, 5 T2, and 2 T3) were suitable for brachytherapy with iridium-192 wire sources [1]. All were N0 at diagnosis and were limited to the glans and/or corona in six, with limited involvement of the shaft in two. Our implants were accomplished using a system similar to that described by Mazeron [23] and detailed below. In our series, 4/8 patients achieved local control with penile preservation. Two experienced local failure and were salvaged by penectomy (one histologically negative). Thus, ultimate local control was achieved in 6 of 8 (75%).

Two patients, the only ones with poorly differentiated lesions, of eight in our series, demonstrated simultaneous local, regional, and distant failure and died with disease. Only 3/45 in Mazeron's series were poorly differentiated, and all but 2/22 in Daly's series were not well differentiated. In Wajman's series [37], however, 20% had high-grade lesions. This relationship of high-grade lesions with poor prognosis has been noted by others [6,7], and more aggressive local regional therapy, even in low-stage disease, should be considered in these cases.

Technique of brachytherapy

Case selection

In general, T1, T2, and limited T3 lesions less than 4 cm in diameter can be considered for implantation, especially in young patients motivated to maintain normal micturition and sexual function. Both local control and preserved function can be achieved in 80% of such cases.

Treatment planning

A single plane of sources is sufficient to encompass small lesions less than 5 mm thick (Figure 1). With more extensive infiltration, at least two planes of implanted sources are required to surround the target volume by the 85% isodose line (Figure 2). Lesions up to 4 cm in diameter can be treated in this

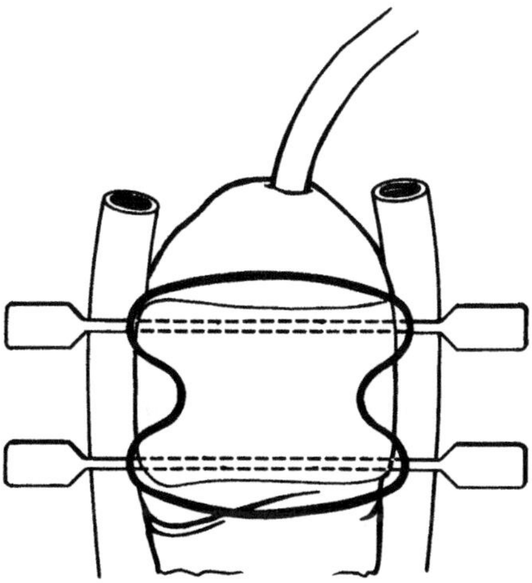

Figure 1. Dorsal view of typical single-plane interstitial implant with the "reference" isodose superimposed (hourglass-shaped heavy black line), which is intended to encompass the tumor target volume.

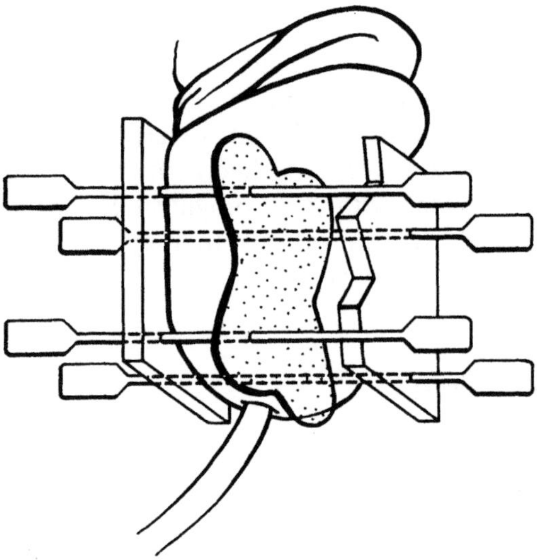

Figure 2. Lateral view of a two-plane implant suitable for a larger tumor than in Figure 1. The outline of the "reference" isodose is indicated by the heavy black line; the plane of the isodose line is stippled.

manner, using up to six sources (Figure 3), which can include tumors originating in the glans with some extension to the cavernous body.

The target tumor dose is 60–65 Gy, delivered at 35–80 cGy/hour in one session, usually requiring 3–4 days. Doses are usually prescribed to the 85% isodose line, the "reference isodose" in the Paris system of dosimetry [2], as described initially by Pierquin and associates. The actual implantation procedure is done under general anesthesia.

After determining the number of iridium-192 sources needed, two lucite templates are prepared with holes predrilled at appropriate locations. Following the templates as a guide, 20- to 22-gauge needles are placed through the penis to surround the lesion (Figure 4), then held in parallel position by the templates. These are secured with lead shot crimped onto the needle points, once everything is properly positioned, and the actual iridium-192 wires have been threaded inside the needles (Figure 5). This partial "afterloading" technique reduces radiation exposure to medical personnel. Following source placement the patient must remain hospitalized in a single bedroom using full radiation protection precautions until the iridium is removed.

Anticipated reactions to treatment

A Foley catheter is kept in place at least for the duration of the implant. Acute mucosal reaction, which peaks by 10–14 days, usually does not require the catheter to remain indwelling and consists of mild to moderate

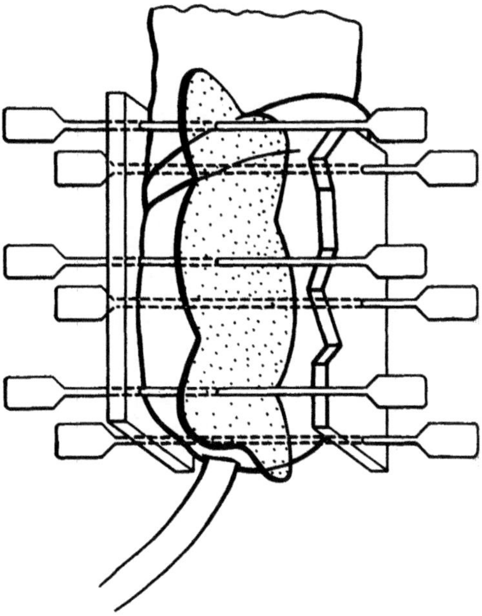

Figure 3. Lateral view of a larger two-plane implant suitable for a tumor with deep infiltration toward the corpora. Note the contraction of the "reference" isodose in the intervals between sources.

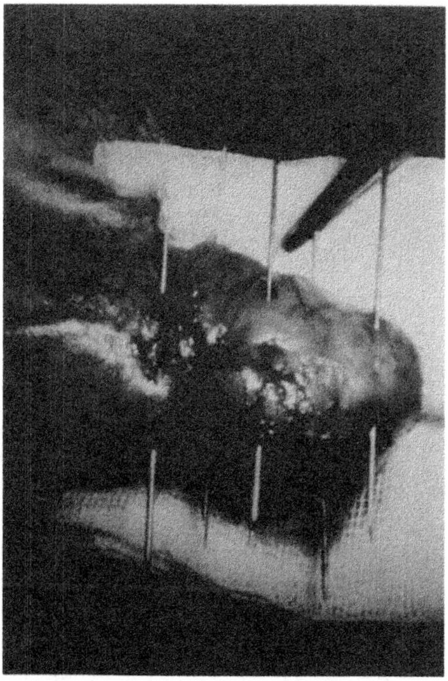

Figure 4. Twenty-gauge needles placed in penis in first plane of planned two-plane implant; both planes will be held in parallel position by templates.

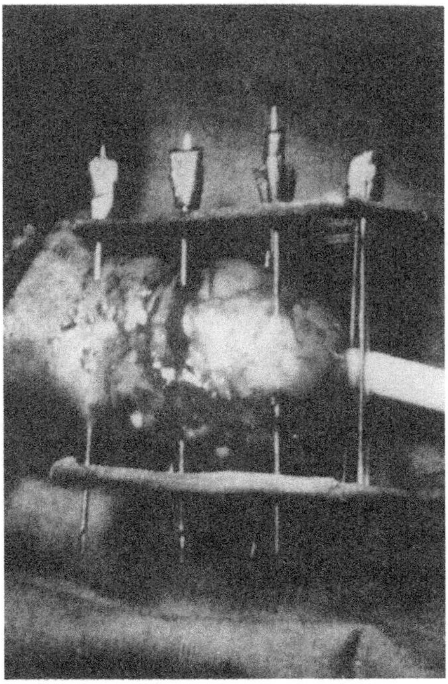

Figure 5. Completed two-plane, six-line implant with templates in place.

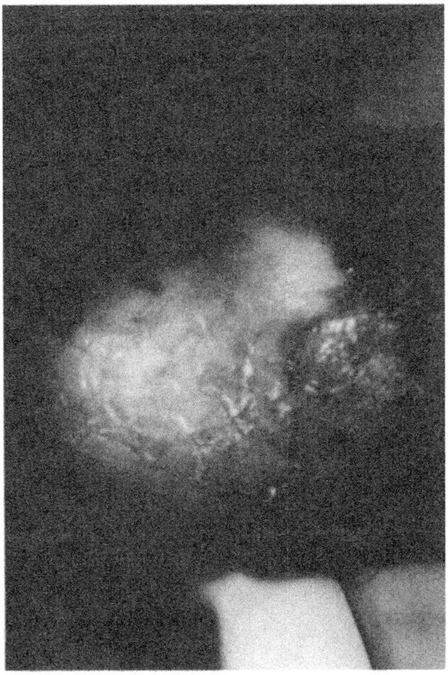

Figure 6. Clinical result at 8 weeks in patient implanted in Figures 4 and 5. Only persistent change is depigmentation. Functional result excellent.

urethral mucosal irritation, which heals over 4–8 weeks, depending on the number or iridium wires implanted. Moderately intense skin reactions appear and heal with about the same time course (Figure 6).

With single plane implants, normal tissue late effects consist mainly of occasional scarring, whereas late reactions are moderate with up to four lines but produce no functional impairment. The risk of necrosis increases with the use of six or more lines. For lesions greater than 4 cm, this risk, as well as the risk of local failure, would favor partial penectomy.

Conclusion

It is apparent that interstitial brachytherapy with iridium-192 wire, using a safe and well-tolerated afterloading technique, can provide effective conservation therapy for selected, early penile carcinomas, with rates of local tumor control comparable to surgical resection. Acute and late sequelae are quite acceptable. Brachytherapy, however, does not impose the major functional or psychological disability associated with partial or total amputation of the penis. It can be anticipated that using iridium-192, 80–90% of suitable patients, namely, those with distal lesions less than 4 cm in diameter, can enjoy local control of tumor with a retained and functional penis.

References

1. Adams PW, Wilson JF: Management of squamous cell carcinoma of the penis: Results of iridium-192 interstitial implantation. Endocuriether/Hypertherm Oncol 6:41–45, 1990.
2. Byhardt R: Penis. In: *Modern Brachytherapy*. Pierquin B, (ed). Wilson JF, Chassagne D (eds). Masson, New York, 1987, pp. 229–232.
3. CA: A Cancer Journal for Physicians, Cancer Statistics, 36(1) 1986.
4. Daly NJ, Douchez J, Combes PF: Treatment of carcinoma of the penis by iridium 192 wire implant. Int J Radiat Oncol Biol Phys 8:1239–1243, 1982.
5. El Demiry MIM, Oliver RTD, Hope-Stone HF, Blandy JP: Reappraisal of the role of radiotherapy and surgery in the management of carcinoma of the penis. Br J Urol 50: 724–728, 1984.
6. Ekstrom T, EdsmyF: Cancer of the penis. A clinical study of 229 cases. Acta Chir Scand 115:25, 1958.
7. Fraley E, Zhang G, Sazama R, Lange PH: Cancer of the penis, prognosis and treatment plans. Cancer 55:1618–1624, 1985.
8. Grabstaldt H, Kelley CD: Radiation of penile cancer. Urology 15:575–576, 1980.
9. Haile K, Delclos L: The place of radiation therapy in the treatment of carcinoma of the distal end of the penis. Cancer 45:1980–1984, 1980.
10. Hanash KA, Furlow WL, Utz DC, Harrison EG: Carcinoma of the penis. A clinicopathologic study. J Urol 104:291, 1970.
11. Harmer MH (ed): *TNM Classification of Malignant Tumors*, 3rd ed. UICC, Geneva, 1978, pp. 126–28.
12. Hasham AI: Autoamputation of the penis from carcinoma. Urology 5:244–245, 1975.
13. Hess F, Prignitz R, Walthers E: Treatment of penis cancer. Urol Int 38:243–246, 1983.
14. Hope-Stone H: Carcinoma of the penis. External radiation mould technique. Proc R Soc Med 68:777–779, 1975.

15. Hoppmann HJ: Diagnosis and management of tumours and tumour like genital lesions. Geriatrics 36:137–142, 1981.
16. Jackson SM: The treatment of cancer of the penis. Br J Surg 53:33–35, 1966.
17. Jensen MS: Cancer of the penis in Denmark 1942 to 1962 (511 cases). Dan Med Bull 24:66–72, 1977.
18. Johnson DE, Fuerst DE, Ayala AG: Carcinoma of the penis; experience with 153 cases. Urology 1:404–408, 1973.
19. Jones WG, Fossa SD, Hamers H, van den Bogaert W: Penis cancer: A review by the Joint Radiotherapy Committee of the European Organisation for Research and Treatment of Cancer (EORTC) Genitourinary and Radiotherapy Groups. J Surg Oncol 40:227–231, 1989.
20. Kaushal V, Sharma SC: Carcinoma of the penis; a 12 year review. Acta Oncolog 26, Fasc. 6, 1987.
21. Knudsen OS, Brennhovd IO: Radiotherapy in the treatment of the primary tumour in penile cancer. Acta Chir Scand 113:69–71, 1967.
22. Krieg RM, Luk KH: Carcinoma of the penis. Review of cases treated by surgery and radiation therapy 1960–1977. Urology 18:149–154, 1981.
23. Mazeron JJ, Langlois D, Lobo PA, Huart JA, Calitchi E, Lusinchi A, Raynal M, Le Bourgeois JP, Abbou CC, Pierquin B: Interstitial radiation therapy for carcinoma of the penis using iridium 192 wires: The Henri Mondor experience (1970–1979). Int J Radiat Oncol Biol Phys 10:1891–1895, 1984.
24. Murrell DS, Williams JL: Radiotherapy in the treatment of carcinoma of the penis. Br J Urol 37:211–222, 1965.
25. Narayana AS, Olney LE, Loening SA, Weimar GW, Culp DA: Carcinoma of the penis, analysis of 219 cases. Cancer 49:2185–2191, 1982.
26. Orr PS, Habeshaw T, Scott R: Carcinoma of the penis: A review of 42 cases. Br J Urol 49:733–738, 1977.
27. Perskey L: Epidemiology of cancer of the penis. In: Grundmann E, Vahlensieck W (eds). *Tumors of the Male Genital System*. Recent Results of Cancer Research, Vol. 60. Springer-Verlag, Berlin, 1977, p. 97.
28. Perskey L, de Kernion J: Carcinoma of the penis. CA 36:258–273, 1986.
29. Pointon RCS: Carcinoma of the penis. External beam therapy. Proc R Soc Med 68: 779–781, 1975.
30. Prassavinichiae S, Schneider H, Brady LW: Carcinoma of the penis. Int J Radiat Oncol Biol Phys 1:1069–1073, 1976.
31. Raynal M, Chassagne D, Baillet F, Pierquin B: Endocurietherapy of penis cancer. In: Grundmann E, Vahlensieck W (eds). *Tumors of the Male Genital System*. Recent Results of Cancer Research, Vol. 60. Springer-Verlag, Berlin, 1977, pp. 135–139.
32. Sagerman RH, Yu WS, Chung CT, Puranik A: External beam irradiation of carcinoma of the penis. Radiology 152:183–185, 1984.
33. Salaverria JC, Hope-Stone HF, Paris AM, Molland EA, Blandy JP: Conservative treatment of carcinoma of the penis. Br J Urol 51:32–37, 1979.
34. Schellhammer PF, Grabstaldt H: Tumors of the penis and urethra. In: Harrison JH, Gittes RF, Perlmutter AD, Stamey TA, Walsh PC (eds). *Campbell's Urology*, Vol. 2, 4th ed. W.B. Saunders, Philadelphia, 1979, pp. 1171–1179.
35. Sharma U, Rath GK, Singhal RM, Sharma LK, Prakash A: Megavoltage radiation therapy in carcinoma of the penis. Int Surg 67:69–71, 1982.
36. Tessler AM, Applebaum SM: The Buschke-Lowenstein tumor. Urology 10:36–39, 1982.
37. Wajsman Z, Moore RH, Merrin CE, Murphy GP: Surgical treatment of penile cancer. Cancer 40:1697–1701, 1977.
38. Yu HHY, Lam P, Leong CH, Ong GB: Carcinoma of the penis; report of 52 cases with reference to lymphography and ilio-inguinal block dissection. Clin Oncol 4:47–53, 1978.

7. Malignancy associated with urinary tract reconstruction using enteric segments

Julia R. Spencer and R. Bruce Filmer

In the last two decades a number of reports of carcinogenesis within enterocystoplasties and conduit urinary diversions have appeared in the literature. Although the numbers are small, characteristics of these tumors are reminiscent of those previously identified in ureterosigmoidostomy patients with anastomotic malignancies. While clinical and experimental data support a role for chemical carcinogens as mediators of tumor formation associated with ureterosigmoidostomy, exposure to a combination of both urinary and fecal streams has traditionally been considered a requirement for the initiation of malignant change. The observation that tumors can occur at or near uroenteric anastomoses in the absence of feces is disturbing and has encouraged a reassessment of the possible pathogenesis of these tumors. Bowel has proven to be a versatile and effective tool in urinary tract reconstruction and has enjoyed a surge in popularity in recent years. Therefore, further clinical and experimental observations are imperative to improve our understanding of why and how often uroenteric tumors occur.

Clinical data

The first clinical use of bowel in reconstruction of the urinary tract, ureterosigmoidostomy, was reported in 1852 [1]. Although initially unsuccessful, the procedure enjoyed increasing popularity after 1920 [2]. The first report of carcinoma at the ureterosigmoidostomy site was published in 1929 [3], but only two more cases were recorded prior to 1960 [4]. Subsequently, however, there was a significant increase in the number of case reports, and a growing concern regarding the risk of this complication is evident in the literature. [2,4,5–8]. The most recent review [2] catalogues 64 reported cases of primary carcinoma (94% adenocarcinoma or "colonic" carcinoma) and 26 cases of adenoma associated with ureterosigmoidostomy; the overall incidence is estimated to be 5–13% [2,4,6,8,9]. The majority occurred at the urocolonic anastomosis, but others arose in the nearby colon or at multiple sites. The latency period varied with the type of tumor and the age of the patient. Carcinoma was diagnosed an average of 25 years

Lepor, H. and Lawson R.K., (eds.), Therapy for Genitourinary Cancer. *ISBN 0-7923-1412-3.*

after diversion [3], while adenomas were diagnosed slightly earlier [10–12]. Younger patients diverted for benign disease presented with tumors on average 25 years postoperatively, while older patients diverted for malignancy exhibited a much shorter mean latency of 10 years [2]. The actual incidence of tumor after ureterosigmoidostomy is difficult to quantitate from these retrospective studies, but there is evidence that it may be higher than initally estimated. Many patients were lost to follow-up, died of other causes, or were undiverted. It would take at least 20 years or more after diversion, and perhaps much longer, to accurately assess risk. Furthermore, colonoscopy screening has detected polyps or dysplasia in as many as 50% of subsets of patients successfully contacted for late follow-up examination [10,13,14]. Although the morphology of these polyps varies, they frequently contain carcinoma in situ and are generally considered premalignant. Biopsies of grossly normal colonic mucosa in patients with ureterosigmoidostomy have revealed abnormal sialomucins, a finding associated with predisposition to colonic carcinoma [9,14–16].

The clinical data show that a finite number of individuals are susceptible to tumorigenesis initiated by one or more carcinogen(s) activated by or present as a result of ureterosigmoidostomy. The long latent interval, appearance of tumors in young patients, cases of multicentricity, and tumors appearing at the anastomotic site long after undiversion [17] all support this assumption. Experimental animal data (*vide infra*) have suggested that an admixture of urine and feces is necessary for malignant change, and urocolonic anastomoses not in contact with the fecal stream were once considered immune to carcinogenesis.

However, in the past 20 years, a number of reports of tumors arising in other forms of uroenteric reconstructions have appeared [18,19]. Malignancies in bladder augmentations have comprised the majority of these cases, and a number of similarities to ureterosigmoidostomy tumors are apparent.

First performed in humans in 1899, enterocystoplasty was popularized after 1950 [20–22]. Ileum was preferred initially, but colo- and cecocystoplasty soon came into general use [23,24]. The first report of an enterocystoplasty tumor appeared in 1971, and a total of 15 cases were reported by 1990 [25–37]. By contrast, 37 years passed before 16 cases of benign and malignant tumors complicating ureterosigmoidostomy were published. The clinical characteristics of enterocystoplasty tumors are listed in Table 1. The majority of procedures were performed for benign disease, primarily tuberculosis. However, vesical tuberculosis without cystoplasty is rarely associated with malignant degeneration [38]. In patients with prior pelvic malignancy, none had evidence of recurrence of that tumor in the augmented bladder. The mean patient age at augmentation was 34 (range 13–49) years, while the mean age at diagnosis of the tumor was 49 (range 42–69) years. The latency interval between augmentation and tumor diagnosis ranged from 5 to 29 years (mean 18 years).

Table 1. Characteristics of patients with neoplasms in enterocystoplasties [25–37] and conduit urinary diversions [43]

	Cystoplasty (n = 15)	Conduit (n = 6)
Original disease		
Tuberculosis	10	—
Exstrophy	—	3
Chronic cystitis	3	—
Neurogenic bladder	1	—
Gynecological cancer	1	2
Unknown	—	1
Enteric segment		
Ileum	10	3
Colon	5	3
Age at tumor (mean, range)	34 (40–69)	40 (23–68)
Latency period (mean, range)	18 (5–29)	13 (1–26)
Tumor position		
At or near uroenteric jcn.	11	3
Enteric segment only	1	3
Bladder only	1	—
Not specified	2	—
Histology		
Adenocarcinoma	10	3
Transitional cell carcinoma	3	—
Adenoma	—	2
Sarcoma	1	—
Oat cell carcinoma	1	—
Anaplastic tumor	—	1
Bacteriuria		
Recurrent	7	1
Documented once	2	1
Not specified	6	4

Of note, 10 of the 15 tumors occurred in ileocystoplasties. This is of concern in view of the rarity of neoplasia in intact ileum [39]. This finding may, however, reflect the earlier preference for ileum in bladder reconstructive surgery. Tumor location was at or near the uroenteric anastomosis in 11 patients, within the enteric segment in one patient, and primarily within the bladder segment in one patient. Data concerning tumor location in the other two patients were not available. Four patients had multifocal lesions.

Adenocarcinoma was the most frequent histologic diagnosis, found in 6 of 9 patients with ileocystoplasty and 4 of 6 patients with colo- or cecocystoplasty. However, a variety of other tumor types occurred. In patients augmented with ileum, two had transitional cell carcinoma with squamous elements and one had undifferentiated sarcoma, while in the colo/cecocystoplasty group, one case each of transitional cell and oat cell carcinoma were described.

Bacteriuria was known to be present in nine patients on at least one occasion; seven had known recurrent urinary tract infection. The remainder of the reports do not include information regarding infection or colonization of the urinary tract. However, bacteriuria is a common finding in patients with enterocystoplasty [20,22,40].

Despite partial or radical cystectomy in 14 patients, four died of disease, seven were alive after a short follow-up (6 months to 3 years) and data were not available for three. One patient died prior to any surgical procedure. Therefore, with only short-term follow-up available, 5 of 15 (33%) patients had already died of their malignancy.

As with enterocystoplasty, ileal conduit urinary diversion was popularized in the 1950s after Bricker's description of the technique [41]. The colon conduit came into general use after 1965 [42]. Six cases of tumor in urinary conduit diversions are listed in the table [43–48]. Other tumors reported in ileal conduits include secondary malignancies and two rare and unusual primary tumors (nephrogenic adenoma [49] and adenocarcinoid tumor [50]) not included in this review.

Of three patients with neoplasms in an ileal conduit, one developed an anaplastic carcinoma with transitional, squamous, and mucin elements 20 years after diversion for exstrophy, at age 28. The tumor was located in the proximal conduit near the uroenteric anastomosis. This patient succumbed to the malignancy. Two other young patients had an adenomatous polyp 15 months and 22 years, respectively, after diversion. One lesion was found in the proximal portion of the conduit and the other was located distally.

All three patients who developed tumors in colon conduits had adenocarcinoma. One occurred in a young patient (age 29) 26 years after diversion and was located near the uroenteric junction. Two other patients in their 60s developed a conduit malignancy 1 and 8 years after diversion required for management of gynecological malignancy. Although the numbers of patients are small, these findings are reminiscent of those seen in ureterosigmoidostomy tumor patients in whom the latency period was shorter in older patients originally diverted because of cancer.

Recurrent bacteriuria was documented in only one patient with a conduit tumor, but bacterial colonization of conduits is known to be quite common, In one study of bacteriuria in urinary diversions, ileal loop urine contained multiple organisms in 73% of cases, while colonic conduit cultures were positive in 37.5% of patients studied, with only a single organism found. [51].

At present, the actual long-term risk of malignant degeneration within urinary conduits and enterocystoplasties is not known. However, while the use of ileum both for conduit diversion and enterocystoplasty has increased since 1950, the data suggest that malignancies are more common in the latter. Possible explanations for this difference include the more extensive uroenteric anastomosis in enterocystoplasty and the longer period of urine storage within the bladder, allowing prolonged exposure of mucosa to putative carcinogens.

Tumor pathogenesis

From the clinical data presented above, we may speculate that uroenteric tumors are the result of one or more carcinogenic stimuli leading to epithelial cell transformation and, after many years, progression to clinically recognized cancer. There is evidence that the process of carcinogenesis occurs in stages, and that different substances and endogenous factors have different roles in the chain of events [52]. Certain substances act as initiators by altering deoxyribonucleic acid structure irreversibly; promoters then reversibly stimulate the growth of the initated cell population, and finally, progression to benign and/or malignant neoplasia occurs via irreversible changes in the cell genome. Some agents are complete carcinogens, able to induce all three phases of malignant transformation. How these principles apply to uroenteric carcinogenesis is completely unknown at present. However, a number of animal studies and observations in humans have provided clues to the possible mechanisms involved.

The majority of animal data pertaining to ureterosigmoidostomy malignancy have been provided by a rat model first described by Crissey and associates [53,54]. Vesicosigmoidostomy with or without proximal diverting colostomy, vesical patch interposition into sigmoid, or sutured colostomy was performed in Wistar Furth rats. Subgroups of rats received bowel and/or bladder carcinogens. Four of six surviving rats with vesicosigmoidostomy that did not receive carcinogen developed polypoid tumors at the anastomosis that appeared to arise from the colon. When urine or feces was diverted away from the uroenteric junction, tumors did not develop. The importance of urine flow past the anastomosis was reiterated by Daher and associates in similar experiments, but only one third of animals developed "adenocarcinoma-like" lesions after vesicosigmoidostomy without proximal fecal diversion [55]. In other studies, animals with interposition of ileum [53] or sigmoid [56] between the uroenteric anastomosis and fecal stream were largely protected from malignancy. Interestingly, in the sigmoid interposition experiments, the tumors that developed did so at the uroenteric anastomosis, not at the junction of urinary and fecal streams (the colo-colonic anastomosis). This observation, and the fact that tumors found in this study were transitional cell type, raises the question of urothelial rather than colonic cell origin. Vesical patches transposed into bowel in other experiments underwent malignant change in 2 of 17 cases (yielding squamous cell carcinoma and adenocarcinoma) [57].

The consensus of data from rat models suggest that direct exposure of a uroenteric anastomosis to both urinary and fecal streams provides the highest risk for carcinogenesis. The most popular theory [58], espoused by many in the last decade, is that formation of N-nitroso compounds by fecal bacterial catalysis of urinary nitrate and secondary amine initiates carcinogenesis in this setting. However, the absence of tumors in Lewis rats subjected to vesicosigmoidostomy, coupled with diminished reactivity to inflammatory stimuli in this strain of rats, suggests that the inflammatory response at the suture line is also important [59], possibly in tumor promotion. Data from animal and human studies in support of these theories are discussed below.

N-nitroso compounds are potent carcinogens that induce tumors in many animal species and that may act as initiators, promoters, or complete carcinogens [60]. However, their activity varies from compound to compound, and the site of experimental tumor formation varies according to species studied, dose, and mode of administration. Some N-nitroso compounds require enzymatic transformation in specific organs in order to form active intermediates, while others do not. The complexities of these compounds with regard to their metabolism, organotropism, and species specificity has made it difficult to determine their role in human cancer or to extrapolate animal data to humans.

However, there is ample evidence that endogenous formation of N-nitroso compounds may occur in humans. Many strains of enterobacteriacae can reduce nitrate to nitrite and catalyze the formation of nitrosamines from nitrite and secondary amine at neutral pH [61–63]. Not present in significant amounts in normal (sterile) urine or in feces, nitrosamines were detected in infected urine from normal [64–67] and augmented [40] bladders and urinary conduits [68] and in rectal slurry specimens after rat or human uroenteric diversion [58,69,70]. Chronic urinary tract infection in rats was associated with early bladder neoplasia [71], and in humans has been linked to bladder cancer in epidemiological studies [72]. Furthermore, urinary infection complicating bladder bilharziasis is theorized to induce carcinogenesis via nitrosamine formation [66,73].

While bacteriuria due to organisms able to catalyze nitrosamine formation is common, the rarity of tumors in this setting suggests that endogenous nitrosation is probably not the sole mediator of uroenteric carcinogenesis. Furthermore, direct evidence linking nitrosamines or other N-nitroso compounds to uroenteric tumors in humans (or in rats) is lacking, and some of the data are conflicting. For example, in the rat ureterosigmoidostomy model, ascorbic acid (known to block nitrosamine formation) [74] did not reduce the incidence of urocolonic tumors in rats, despite a significant reduction in measured nitrosamine [75]. A recent study, in which strict analytical methodology was used, reported significantly higher levels of N-nitroso compounds in humans, but not in rats, after ureterosigmoidostomy compared to controls [70]. These authors suggested that factors other than N-nitrosation are important in the pathogenesis of urocolonic tumors.

The inflammatory response itself may be important in the pathogenesis of uroenteric tumors, occurring in response to sutures, infection, and/or chronic irritation. For example, inflammation and hyperplasia may play a role in cancers occurring in catheterized, chronically infected spinal cord injury patients [76] or in suture-line recurrences of colon carcinoma [77]. Histological studies of urinary conduits and cystoplasties have demonstrated frequent, often severe, chronic inflammatory changes, especially in long-standing diversions [15,40,78,79]. Although not premalignant per se, the inflammatory process may, in concert with other factors, contribute to malignant change in some individuals. In animals, chemical carcinogenesis is enhanced by surgical incisions or suture in colon or bladder [80,81]. Persistant increased cell proliferation near colonic anastomoses, despite complete healing, was associated with an increased susceptibility to carcinogens, even 3 months after surgery [81].

Activated macrophages may play a role in carcinogenesis, either by production of reactive oxygen species [82] or by synthesis of nitrate, nitrite, and nitrosamine [83]. Inflammatory cells also produce growth factors, which may act as promoters in the process of malignant transformation [84]. Epidermal growth factor (EGF) is a constituent of the urinary fraction that enhances carcinogen-induced bladder carcinoma in rats [85]. Therefore, EGF produced by inflammatory cells or present in urine may contribute to carcinogenesis.

Variation in the degree of inflammatory response may explain individual differences in tumor susceptibility. Studies of Lewis rats, resistant to vesicosigmoidostomy tumors, have shown that superoxide production by activated macrophages and urinary nitrate excretion in response to inflammation is significantly lower in this strain of rats than in those prone to urocolonic tumors [59].

One measure of proliferative activity that may be a specific predictor of cancer promotion is ornithine decarboxylase, an intracellular enzyme that catalyzes polyamine biosynthesis. Induction of the enzyme is correlated with tumor-promoting activity and is observed in experimental bladder carcinogenesis [86], as well as in association with ureterosigmoidostomy [87] and colonic neoplasia [88]. Also, α-difluoromethylornithine, an inhibitor of ornithine decarboxylase, can inhibit the formation of nitrosamine-induced rat bladder tumors [89].

It is likely that more than one factor is responsible for uroenteric malignancy, and it is possible that more than one mechanism was operative in the cases presented herein. One or more carcinogen(s), perhaps not yet identified, may initiate the process within transitional or enteric epithelium; tumor promotion may be mediated by endogenous bacterial nitrosation, inflammation, growth factors, or other urinary constituents; and, in some patients, progression to invasive cancer may occur.

Patient surveillance

Although the actual long-term risk of tumor degeneration in uroenteric reconstructions is unknown and the etiology remains speculative, it appears that a small but finite number of patients are at risk. Therefore, long-term follow-up of all patients with enteric segments in the urinary tract is mandatory to better assess the incidence of malignancy and to allow earlier intervention.

Standard imaging studies (intravenous urography, ultrasound, cystography) are probably not sufficiently sensitive to allow the early diagnosis of cystoplasty tumors. Urinary cytological examination, particularly when specimen collection is aided by bladder barbottage, is probably useful, although not yet tested in this setting. However, the interpretation of cytology specimens may be impeded in some cases by the presence of chronic infection and/or inflammation [90]. Certainly, these patients should undergo periodic urinary cytologic examination, but it is unclear at this time if cytology alone is adequate for long-term follow-up.

Endoscopy with biopsy, as warranted, may be the most sensitive method of surveillance in cystoplasty patients. For example, areas of dysplasia or benign polypoid lesions may be diagnosed in patients with negative urinary cytology results. Periodic examinations should begin by 10 years after surgery (perhaps earlier in older patients, especially those with colon augmentations), and the frequency of follow-up should be dictated by findings. Cases in which preexisting enteric conduits were incorporated into the augmentation or with preexisting bladder exstrophy should be examined earlier and more frequently.

Patients with enteric conduits probably do not require such close surveillance. However, in older patients, preoperative barium enema or (preferably) colonoscopy is advisable if colonic conduit diversion is planned. The elderly also merit closer postoperative follow-up in view of their higher risk for spontaneous colon carcinoma.

Possible preventive measures in uroenteric malignancy are only theoretical at this time. Correlation of the type and incidence of bacteriuria with long-term risk for neoplasia would be useful, but effective eradication of organisms, particularly in cystoplasty patients undergoing clean intermittent catheterization, is unlikely. Future comprehensive experiments should be undertaken to evaluate the usefulness of other chemopreventive agents in animal models. Finally, a trend toward alternative techniques for urinary tract reconstruction, particularly in children, should be encouraged.

Conclusions

Based on data available to date, certain uroenteric reconstructions appear to carry a small but definite risk of malignant degeneration. Carcinogenesis in ureterosigmoidostomy and cystoplasty is much more common than in ileal conduit diversion, despite widespread use of the latter. It is too early to assess the risk for malignancy in colonic conduits, continent diversions, and bladder substitutions using bowel, since these procedures have been popular for less than 20 years. Tumor etiology is unknown but probably multifactorial. Despite speculation that urinary N-nitroso compound formation is responsible for tumorigenesis, there are no firm data to support this impression. Tumor histology so far has been variable, and it is not known whether tumors arise from transitional or enteric epithelium. Despite the lack of data regarding the incidence and pathogenesis, the increasing number of cases and the observation that these tumors are quite capable of aggressive behavior is worrisome. Therefore, a high index of suspicion and close, long-term follow-up of all patients with uroenteric reconstructions is warranted.

References

1. Simon J: Ectopia vesicae (absence of the anterior walls of the bladder and pubic abdominal pareites): Operation for directing the orifices of the ureters into the rectum. Temporary success: subsequent death: autopsy. Lancet 2:568, 1852.
2. Stewart M: Urinary diversion and bowel cancer. Ann R Coll Surg Engl 68:98–102, 1986.
3. Hammer E: Cancer du colon sigmoide dix ans apres implantation des ureteres d'une vessie exstrophiée. J Urol (Paris) 28:260–263, 1929.
4. Urdaneta LF, Duffell D, Creevy CD, Aust JB: Late development of primary carcinoma of the colon following ureterosigmoidostomy: Report of 3 cases and literature review. Ann Surg 164:503–513, 1966.
5. Whitaker RE, Pugh RCB, Dow D: Colonic tumors following ureterosigmoidostomy. Br J Urol 43:562–575, 1971.
6. Parsons CD, Thomas MH, Garrett RA: Colonic adenocarcinoma: A delayed complication of ureterosigmoidostomy. J Urol 118:31–34, 1977.
7. Spence HM, Hoffman WW, Rosmire GP: Tumour of the colon as a late complication of ureterosigmoidostomy for exstrophy of the bladder. Br J Urol 51:466–470, 1979.
8. Leadbetter GW, Zickerman P, Pierce E: Ureterosigmoidostomy and carcinoma of the colon. J Urol 121:732–735, 1979.
9. Silverman SH, Woodhouse CRJ, Strachan JR, Cumming J, Keighley MRB: Long-term management of patients who have had urinary diversions into colon. Br J Urol 58:634–639, 1986.
10. Stewart M, Macrae FA, Williams CB: Neoplasia and ureterosigmoidostomy: A colonoscopy survey. Br J Surg 69:414–416, 1982.
11. Ali MH, Satti MB, Al-Nafussi A: Multiple benign colonic polypi at the site of ureterosigmoidostomy. Cancer 53:1006–1010, 1984.
12. VanDriel MF, Zwiers W, Grond J, Verschueren RCJ, Mensink HJA: Juvenile polyps at the site of a ureterosigmoidostomy. Dis Colon Rectum 31:553–557, 1988.
13. Starling JR, Uehling DT, Gilchrist KW: Value of colonoscopy after ureterosigmoidostomy. Surgery 96:784–789, 1984.
14. Gilchrist KW, Uehling DT, Starling JR: Cancer surveillance after ureterosigmoidostomy: Colonic microscopic changes. J Surg Res 36:251–255, 1984.
15. Tomasino RM, Morello V, Latteri MA, Spinnato G, Pantuso G, Orestano R: Histological and histochemical changes in the colon mucosa after ureterosigmoidostomy or colonic conduit. Eur Urol 15:248–251, 1988.
16. Marcheggiano A, Iannoni C, Pallone F, Frieri G, Galluci M, Caprilli R: Abnormal patterns of colonic mucin secretion after ureterosigmoidostomy. Hum Pathol 15:647–650, 1984.
17. Sohn M, Füzesi L, Deutz F, LaGrange W, Kirkpatrick JC, Braun JC: Signet ring cell carcinoma in adenomatous polyp at site of ureterosigmoidostomy 16 years after conversion to ileal conduit. J Urol 143:805–807, 1990.
18. Harzmann R: Harnableitungskarzinom — Fiktion oder Realitat? Akt Urol 20:179–183, 1989.

19. Filmer RB, Spencer JR: Malignancies in bladder augmentations and intestinal conduits. J Urol 143:671–678, 1990.
20. Goodwin WE, Turner RD, Winter CC: Results of ileocystoplasty. J Urol 80:461–466, 1958.
21. Küss R, Bitker M, Camey M, Chatelain C, Lassau JP: Indications and early and late results of intestino-cystoplasty: A review of 185 cases. J Urol 103:53–63, 1970.
22. Dounis A, Gow JG: Bladder augmentation: A long-term review. Br J Urol 51:264–268, 1979.
23. Winter CC, Goodwin WE: Results of sigmoidocystoplasty. J Urol 80:467–472, 1958.
24. Charghi A, Charbonneau J, Gauthier GE: Colocystoplasty for bladder enlargement and substitution: A study of late results in 31 cases. J Urol 97:849–856, 1967.
25. Smith P, Hardy GJ: Carcinoma occurring as a late complication of ileocystoplasty. Br J Urol 43:576–579, 1971.
26. Leedham PW, England HR: Adenocarcinoma developing in an ileocystoplasty. Br J Surg 60:158–160, 1973.
27. Egbert BM, Kraft JK, Perkash I: Undifferentiated sarcoma arising in an augmented ileocystoplasty patch. J Urol 123:272–274, 1980.
28. Takasaki E, Murahashi I, Toyoda M, Honda M, Waku S: Signet ring adenocarcinoma of ileal segment following ileocystoplasty. J Urol 130:562–563, 1983.
29. Kamidono S, Arakawa S, Umezu K, Ishigami J, Maeda S: A rare case of adenocarcinoma of bladder following augmentation enterocystoplasty. Acta Urol Jpn 31:315–318, 1985.
30. Kirby RS, Lloyd-Davies RW: Adenocarcinoma occurring within a caecocystoplasty. Br J Urol 57:357–358, 1985.
31. Steg A, Conquy S, Teyssier P, Amar E, Schrameck E, Boiteux JP: Colonic adenocarcinoma arising after uretero-sigmoidostomy or after bladder enlargement by a colonic segment. Ann Urol 19:283–287, 1985.
32. Stone AR, Stephenson TP: Tumors associated with lower tract reconstruction using isolated bowel segments. In: King LR, Stone AR, Webster GD (eds). *Bladder Reconstruction and Continent Urinary Diversion*. Year Book Medical Publishers, Chicago, 1987, pp. 93–98.
33. Hasegawa S, Ohshima S, Kinukawa T, Matsuura O, Takeuchi Y, Hattori R, Murakami S: Adenocarcinoma of the bladder 29 years after ileocystoplasty. Br J Urol 61:162–167, 1988.
34. Harzmann R, Kopper B, Carl P: Karzinomin duktion durch Harnab-oder-umleitung uber Darmabschnitte? Urologe A 25:198–203, 1986.
35. Grainger R, Kenny A, Walsh A: Adenocarcinoma of the caecum occurring in a caecocystoplasty. Br J Urol 61:164–165, 1988.
36. Golomb J, Klutke CG, Lewin KJ, Goodwin WE, deKernion JB, Raz S: Bladder neoplasms associated with augmentation cystoplasty: Report of 2 cases and literature review. J Urol 142:377–380, 1989.
37. Kadow C, Heaton ND, Pues T, Yates-Bell AJ, Packham DA: Adenocarcinoma in a substitution caecocystoplasty. Br J Urol 63:649–650, 1989.
38. Takayama K, Kumazawa J, Minoda K: Bladder tumor occurring in the contracted bladder following urinary tract tuberculosis. Eur Urol 12:448–450, 1986.
39. Perzin KH, Bridge MF: Adenomas of the small intestine: A clinicopathologic review of 51 cases and a study of their relationship to carcinoma. Cancer 48:799–819, 1981.
40. Nurse DE, Mundy AR: Assessment of the malignant potential of cystoplasty. Br J Urol 64:489–492, 1989.
41. Bricker EM: Bladder substitution after pelvic evisceration. Surg Clin North Am 30: 1511–1521, 1950.
42. Mogg RA: The treatment of neurogenic urinary incontinence using the colonic conduit. Br J Urol 37:681–686, 1965.
43. Shousa S, Scott J, Polak J: Ileal loop carcinoma after cystectomy for bladder exstrophy. Br Med J 2:397–398, 1978.
44. Tomera KM, Unni KK, Utz DC: Adenomatous polyp in ileal conduit. J Urol 128: 1025–1026, 1982.

45. Peterson NE: Adenoma of ileal urinary conduit. J Urol 131:1171–1172, 1984.
46. Chiang MS, Minton JP, Clausen K, Clatworthy HW, Wise HA: Carcinoma in a colon conduit urinary diversion. J Urol 127:1185–1187, 1982.
47. Wilson JWL, Morales A: Development of adenocarcinoma in transverse colon conduit. Urology 20:182–183, 1982.
48. Marchetti DL, Piver MS, Tsukada Y: Adenocarcinoma in an isolated sigmoid urinary conduit. Obstet Gynecol 63 (Suppl. 3):54S–56S, 1984.
49. Strand WR, Alfert HJ: Nephrogenic adenoma occurring in an ileal conduit. J Urol 137:491–492, 1987.
50. Kochevar J: Adenocarcinoid tumor, goblet cell type, arising in a ureteroileal conduit: A case report. J Urol 131:957–959, 1984.
51. Hill MJ, Hudson MJ, Stewart M: The urinary bacterial flora in patients with 3 types of urinary tract diversion. J Med Microbiol 16:221–226, 1983.
52. Pitot HC: Mechanisms of chemical carcinogenesis: Theoretical and experimental bases. In: Cooper CS, Grover PL (eds). *Chemical Carcinogenesis and Mutagenesis I*. Springer-Verlag, Berlin, 1990, pp. 3–29.
53. Crissey MM, Steele GD, Gittes RF: Rat model for carcinogenesis in ureterosigmoidostomy. Science 207:1079–1080, 1980.
54. Crissey MM, Steele GD, Gittes RF: Ureterosigmoidostomy and colon carcinogenesis (letter). Science 214:351, 1981.
55. Daher N, Gautier R, Abourachid H, Decaens C, Bara J: Rat colonic carcinogenesis after ureterosigmoidostomy: Pathogenesis and immunohistochemical study. J Urol 139: 1331–1336, 1988.
56. Shands C, McDougal WS, Wright EP: Prevention of cancer at the urothelial enteric anastomotic site. J Urol 141:178–181, 1989.
57. Aaronson IA, Constantinides CG, Sallie LP, Sinclair-Smith CC: Pathogenesis of adenocarcinoma complicating ureterosigmoidostomy: Experimental observations. Urology 29: 538–543, 1987.
58. Stewart M, Hill MJ, Pugh RCB, Williams JP: The role of N-nitrosamine in carcinogenesis at the ureterocolic anastomosis. Br J Urol 53:115–118, 1981.
59. Dull BJ, Gittes RF, Goldman P: Nitrate production and phagocyte activation; Differences among Sprague-Dawley, Wistar-Furth and Lewis rats. Carcinogenesis 9:625–627, 1988.
60. Lawley PD: N-nitroso compounds. In: Cooper CS, Grover PL (eds). *Chemical Carcinogenesis and Mutagenesis II*. Springer-Verlag, Berlin, 1990, pp. 411–469.
61. Hawksworth GM, Hill MJ: Bacterial and the N-nitrosation of secondary amines. Br J Cancer 25:520–526, 1971.
62. Leach SA, Cook AR, Challis BC, Hill MJ, Thompson MH: Bacterially mediated N-nitrosation reactions and endogenous formation of N-nitroso compounds. In: Bartsch H, O'Neill IK, Schulte-Hermann R (eds). *Relevance of N-Nitroso Compounds to Human Cancer: Exposures and Mechanisms*. IARC Scientific Publications, Lyon, No. 84, 1987, pp. 396–399.
63. Calmels S, Ohshima H, Vincent P, Gounot AM, Bartsch H: Screening of microorganisms for nitrosation catalysis at pH 7 and kinetic studies on nitrosamine formation from secondary amines by *E. coli* strains. Carcinogenesis 6:911–915, 1985.
64. Davis CP, Cohen MS, Anderson MD, Gruber MB, Warren MM: Urothelial hyperplasia and neoplasia. II. Detection of nitrosamines and interferon in chronic urinary tract infections in rats. J Urol 134:1002–1006, 1985.
65. Ohshima H, Calmels S, Pignatelli B, Vincent P, Bartsch H: N-nitrosamine formation in urinary-tract infections. In: Bartsch H, O'Neill IK, Schulte-Hermann R (eds). *Relevance of N-Nitroso Compounds to Human Cancer: Exposures and Mechanisms*. IARC Scientific Publications, Lyon, No. 84, 1987, pp. 384–390.
66. Hicks RM, Walters CL, Elsebai I, El-Aaser A-B, El-Merzabani M, Gough TA: Demonstration of nitrosamines in human urine: Preliminary observations on a possible etiology for bladder cancer in association with chronic urinary tract infections. Proc R Soc Med 70: 413–417, 1977.

67. Radomski JL, Greenwald D, Hearn WL, Block NL, Woods FM: Nitrosamine formation in bladder infections and its role in the etiology of bladder cancer. J Urol 120:48–50, 1978.
68. Tricker AR, Kälble T, Preussmann R: Increased urinary nitrosamine excretion in patients with urinary diversions. Carcinogenesis 10:2379–2382, 1989.
69. Cohen MS, Hilz ME, Davis CP, Anderson MD: Urinary carcinogen (nitrosamine) production in a rat animal model for ureterosigmoidostomy. J Urol 138:449–452, 1987.
70. Kälble T, Tricker AR, Mohring K, Berger MR, Geiss H, Staehler G: The role of nitrate, nitrite and N-nitrosamines in carcinogenesis of colon tumours following ureterosigmoidostomy. Urol Res 18:123–129, 1990.
71. Davis CP, Cohen MS, Gruber MB, Anderson MD, Warren MM: Urothelial hyperplasia and neoplasia: A response to chronic urinary tract infections in rats. J Urol 132:1025–1031, 1984.
72. Kantor AF, Hartge P, Hoover RN, Narayana AS, Sullivan JW, Fraumeni JF: Urinary tract infection and risk of bladder cancer. Am J Epidemiol 119:510–515, 1984.
73. Tricker AR, Mostafa MK, Spiegelhalder B, Preussman R: Urinary excretion of nitrate, nitrite and N-nitroso compounds in Schistosomiasis and bilharzia bladder cancer patients. Carcinogenesis 10:547–552, 1989.
74. Mirvish SS, Walcave L, Eagen M, Shubik P: Ascorbate-nitrate reaction: Possible means of blocking the formation of carcinogenic N-nitroso compounds. Science 177:65–68, 1972.
75. Stribling MD, Cohen MS, Fagan JD, Sanchez RL, Anderson MD, Davis CP, Warren MM: The effect of ascorbic acid on urinary nitrosamines and tumor development in a rat animal model for ureterosigmoidostomy (abstr). J Urol 141:304A, 1989.
76. Kaufman JM, Fam B, Jacobs SC, Gabilondo F, Yalla S, Kane JP, Rossier AB: Bladder cancer and squamous metaplasia in spinal cord injury patients. J Urol 118:967–971, 1977.
77. Keighley MRB, Hall C: Anastomotic recurrence of colon cancer — a biological phenomenon or an avoidable calamity? Gut 28:786–791, 1987.
78. Moorcraft J, DuBoulay CEH, Isaacson P, Atwell JD: Changes in the mucosa of colon conduits with particular reference to the risk of malignant change. Br J Urol 55:185–188, 1983.
79. Deane AM, Woodhouse CRJ, Parkinson MC: Histological changes in ileal conduits. J Urol 132:1108–1111, 1984.
80. Chester JF, Gaissert HA, Ross JS, Malt RA, Weitzman SA: N-[4-(5-nitro-2-furyl)-2-thiazolyl] formamide-induced bladder cancer in mice: Augmentation by sutures through the bladder wall. J Urol 137:769–771, 1987.
81. Roe R, Fermor B, Williamson RCN: Proliferative instability and experimental carcinogenesis at colonic anastomoses. Gut 28:808–815, 1987.
82. Weitzman SA, Weitberg AB, Clark EP, Stossel TP: Phagocytes as carcinogens: Malignant transformation produced by human neutrophils. Science 227:1231–1233, 1985.
83. Iyengar R, Stuehr DJ, Marletta MA: Macrophage synthesis of nitrite, nitrate and N-nitrosamines: Precursors and role of the respiratory burst. Proc Natl Acad Sci USA 84:6369–6373, 1987.
84. Sporn MB, Roberts AB: Peptide growth factors and inflammation, tissue repair, and cancer. J Clin Invest 78:329–332, 1986.
85. Yura Y, Hayashi O, Kelly M, Oyasu R: Identification of epidermal growth factor as a component of the rat urinary bladder tumor-enhancing urinary fractions. Cancer Res 49:1548–1553, 1989.
86. Babaya K, Izumi K, Ozono S, Miyata Y, Morikawa A, Chmiel JS, Oyasu R: Capability of urinary components to enhance ornithine decarboxylase activity and promote urothelial tumorigenicity. Cancer Res 43:1774–1782, 1983.
87. Weber TR, Westfall SH, Steinhardt GF, Webb L, Sotelo-Avila C, Connors RH: Malignancy associated with ureterosigmoidostomy: Detection by mucosa ornithine decarboxylase. J Ped Surg 23:1091–1094, 1988.
88. Moorehead RJ, Hoper M, McKelvey STD: Assessment of ornithine decarboxylase activity in rectal mucosa as a marker for colorectal adenomas and carcinomas. Br J Surg 74: 364–365, 1987.

89. Homma Y, Kakizoe T, Samma S, Oyasu R: Inhibition of N-butyl-N-(4-hydroxybutyl)nitrosamine-induced rat urinary bladder carcinogenesis by α-difluoromethylornithine. Cancer Res 47:6176–6179, 1987.
90. deVoogt HD, Rather P, Beyer-Boon ME: Urinary Cytology. Springer-Verlag, New York, 1977, pp. 55–61.

8. Evolving concepts in surgical management of testis cancer

John P. Donohue, Richard Bihrle and Richard S. Foster

Nonseminomatous germ cell tumor is an extraordinary tumor in terms of demonstrating the impact of regional lymphadenectomy on survival. Over the years many series have shown that node-positive (pathologic stage II) patients can still be cured with local measures in excess of 50% of the time. There are a variety of anatomical considerations that make testicular lymphatic drainage predictable. These relate to features of anatomic descent of the gonad and its associated lymphatics. A number of topographic studies have supported the regional deposition of metastatic disease, and we have a good understanding of this. More importantly, there are biologic considerations that probably lend to the opportunity for cure with testis cancer patients with surgery alone. Many patients will have teratomatous elements that have somewhat lower metastatic potential. What is fascinating, however, is that even undifferentiated germ cell tumors, such as embryonal cancer, still are often cured with lymphadenectomy alone. Data recently presented in the *New England Journal of Medicine* in the cooperative multi-institutional study show that a control group treated with node dissection alone had more than half of the patients as long-term survivors without relapse [1].

Fortunately, the relapsers were rescued at the time of relapse, with only a few exceptions. The overall survival in Stage II disease, including all levels of involvement (both Stage II-A and II-B) is 97.5%. Naturally, this has been achieved with the use of either adjuvant chemotherapy immediately following RPLND or full-course chemotherapy, given only at the time of relapse, in the other half of patients, who relapsed after earlier RPLND and were observed only for Stage II disease.

A general treatment philosophy when considering retroperitoneal node dissections should be as follows: The surgery should be appropriate (let the punishment fit the crime). Although presently our position in low-stage low-volume disease is divergent from those committed to surveillance only, I see our paths converging. Clearly, no one wants to do staging RPLND for its own sake. If we can get the sensitivity of clinical staging at levels of confidence exceeding the 90% percentile, there will be no need to do staging RPLNDs. In the meantime, however, a good interim position is the

Lepor, H. and Lawson R.K., (eds.), Therapy for Genitourinary Cancer.
Kluwer Academic Publishers. ISBN 0-7923-1412-3.

modified RPLND, particularly that employing nerve-sparing techniques. Virtually all patients who have a nerve-sparing modified RPLND will ejaculate. Hence, the patient has not been harmed, and he has also been adequately staged. In fact, those who do have microscopic disease have also been given a therapeutic procedure. At this point the relapse rate locally in patients with nervesparing RPLND is entirely satisfactory in our current small and selected series [2].

Regarding high-stage disease, our reviews are generally concordant with other groups throughout the world. Disseminated disease requires disseminated treatment first. This implies pretreatment with systemic chemotherapy that is platinum based. Currently programs employing platinum VP-16, with or without bleomycin, are quite popular and effective. Surgery is reserved for those who have residual clinical disease as noted on the CT scan. One of our current challenges is to see if we can develop predictive criteria for those who might have scar tissue and necrosis only in the specimen. There is some analogy with the seminoma data for advanced disease, where it has been found that most patients with a partical remission can be followed because they will have necrosis only in their tissue specimen. However, there are always exceptions to the rule, and they must be followed carefully, and relapse must be treated aggressively when and if it occurs.

Another philosophical point that will impact the future management of node dissection in testis cancer is that health care providers will want to eliminate qualitative variables in treatment programs as much as possible. Surgery is always a variable in this regard. In order to simplify and codify quantitative aspects of treatment, there will be a move to eliminate initial hospital costs in such things as staging and/or treatment for low-stage disease. Systemic chemotherapy is more easily standardized and quantified. Surgery for low-volume disease, therefore, may be dismantled, except in a salvage setting. Unfortunately, this will require many patients with low-volume disease limited to the retroperitoneum to undergo a highly toxic program that may well have negative long-term consequences on their fertility. Primary germ cell damage is well known in our treatment for advanced disease, and only about half of our patients regenerate a satisfactory sperm count after 2 or 3 years. Hopefully this will not become a treatment excess for low-volume disease patients in the future. It seems a good deal simpler and more direct to treat low-volume disease surgically and to eliminate the potential of local relapse in an area (retroperitoneum) difficult to monitor and follow.

My own view is that surgery should be more proactive than reactive in the treatment of low-stage disease. Surgery can cure the malignant process literally in hours. When it does not, a cure is then available, should the patient relapse, almost always in a pulmonary mode, which is easily detectable and treatable. Again, this is the only solid tumor that is curable by surgery alone more than 50% of the time when the regional nodes are positive. So, the approach to the retroperitoneum is even more feasible and less toxic longterm with the development of anatomical nerve-sparing dissections, which will preserve ejaculation. At least this gives us an option to surveillance, which seems to be quite effective and reasonable.

Finally, concerning high-stage disease, there is general agreement that all persistent tumors, after initial chemotherapy, should be removed. We have noted that certain patients with very favorable response criteria can be followed with the expectation of further resolution of their radiographic changes [3]. Our hope is that we can be more selective in choosing patients for postchemotherapy surgery. In the meantime, however, if there is any significant concern about the presence of persistent tumor, as a general principle such patients are more safely managed with exploration and RPLND. Currently with this approach in over 300 postchemotherapy RPLNDs, we have 44% with necrosis/fibrosis only, 44% with teratoma, and 12% with cancer. The former two groups are carefully observed postoperatively, and the last group with persistent cancer receives two courses of salvage chemotherapy. The overall survival of this group is good (80–90%), but factors predicting for relapse are bulk of tumor, histology, and site (primary mediastinum) [4, 5].

Surgery for massive metastatic disease in testis cancer has become reasonable and appropriate in view of the great advances in chemotherapy for advanced disease [6]. The majority of patients will have their bulky disease reduced in volume and also downgraded histologically into a more mature teratomatous or even necrotic form. Of course, some persist with malignant elements as well [4–12].

From a medical oncologic viewpoint, this is critical information because it will guide subsequent medical management. Those with persistent malignant tumor require further salvage chemotherapy. Those with only teratoma or necrosis in the specimen will be managed expectantly.

Often these retroperitoneal tumors are massive. It is of vital importance to resect them completely, because local or regional recurrence is quite possible, particularly in the more extensive bulky tumors. Hence, this area represents one of the ultimate surgical challenges. Total tumor extirpation is required with exceptional demands on vascular isolation and preservation. Aggressive ablative purpose must be combined with thoughtful and delicate dissection.

Rationale and results of nerve-sparing retroperitoneal lymphadenectomy in clinical stage I testis cancer

The rationale for the use of retroperitoneal lymphadenectomy in low-stage testis cancer is well grounded. Retroperitoneal lymphadenectomy in this situation is useful in terms of staging because approximately 30% of patients with clinical stage A testis cancer, indeed, are pathologic stage B. In addition, testis cancer is unusual in that removal of metastatic disease from the retroperitoneum is curative in 50–80% of cases [1]. Hence, the usefulness of retroperitoneal lymphadenectomy in low-stage nonseminomatous testicular carcinoma is twofold: staging and therapeutic.

The major objection to retroperitoneal lymphadenectomy in low-stage nonseminomatous carcinoma of the testis has been the fertility consequences of lymphadenectomy. Patients who undergo full bilateral lymphadenectomy universally lose emission and the ability to ejaculate [13]. This major source of morbidity has been the impetus for the development of surveillance protocols.

With the development of more effective treatment for nonseminomatous testis cancer, the issue of morbidity of treatment has become more important. These young men now are likely to be cured of their disease and demand the same quality of life as their peers. Therefore, the concept of preserving ejaculatory ability without compromising the efficacy of the procedure became an important one.

Nodal distribution studies in nonseminomatous testis cancer afforded an understanding of the likely sites of retroperitoneal metastasis in low-volume disease [11]. So-called modified retroperitoneal lymph node dissections were developed with these mapping studies in mind. Only the lymphatic tissue possessing a high probability of retroperitoneal metastasis was removed, with other lymphatic tissue being left intact. These modified techniques yielded a preservation of emission/ejaculation at approximately the 70% level. This was a definite advancement in the reducing the morbidity of therapy of this disease. However, with increasing knowledge of the anatomy of the sympathetic nervous system in the retroperitoneum, investigators questioned whether or not ejaculatory ability could be preserved 100% of the time without compromising the efficacy of the operation. We describe the results from Indiana University of the first 75 patients to undergo prospective nerve-sparing retroperitoneal lymphadenectomy in low-stage nonseminomatous carcinoma of the testis.

Patients presenting with a diagnosis of nonseminomatous carcinoma of the testis post radical orchiectomy were subjected to clinical staging consisting of abdominal and chest computed tomography and determination of serum alpha-fetoprotein and beta-HCG. Patients who had normal CT scans of the abdomen and chest, an either normal markers or markers falling on the normal decay curve, were considered candidates for nerve-sparing lymphadenectomy.

A midline transperitoneal approach is utilized. After opening the abdomen initially, the retroperitoneum and nodal tissue along the internal spermatic vessels are palpated. If indeed clinical staging was accurate and no adenopathy is palpated, nerve-sparing retroperitoneal lymphadenectomy is performed. The posterior peritoneal incisions for nerve-sparing lymphadenectomy are somewhat limited compared to the incision utilized for full bilateral lymphadenectomy.

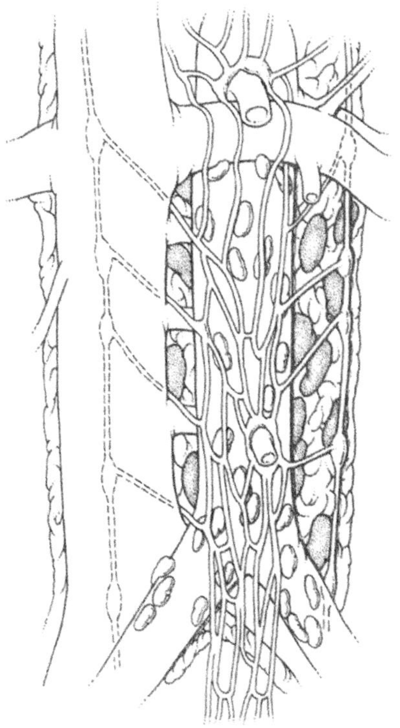

Figure 1. Anterior view of relationships of postganglionic fibers of L-1 through L-4 to the great vessels. The right sympathetic chain is dorsal to the vena cava, with its post ganglionic branches emerging posteromedially to decussate with the hypogastric plexus of nerves anterior to the aorta. Several trunks then course anterior to the iliac vessels into the true pelvis.

For a right-sided dissection, an incision is made in the posterior peritoneum from approximately the cecum cephalad to the area of the ligament of Treitz (Figure 1). Blunt and sharp dissection are then utilized to elevate the root of the small bowel off the lymphatic tissue and great vessels, exposing the interaortacaval, precaval, and right pericaval zones. Self-retaining retractors are useful in order to provide adequate exposure. The split and roll technique is used to divide the lymphatic tissue overlying the vena cava after careful palpation has disclosed no precaval renal arteries. This lymphatic tissue is then rolled off the vena cava both medially and laterally. Medially in the interaortacaval zone, close inspection will reveal sympathetic fibers coursing from the sympathetic chain around lumbar veins into the interaortacaval zone and caudally to the bifurcation of the aorta (Figure 2). These fibers are identified and dissected free of lymphatic tissue prior to the lymphadenectomy. After the prospective dissection of these fibers, lymphatic tissue is removed according to the standard templates dictated by mapping studies (Figure 3).

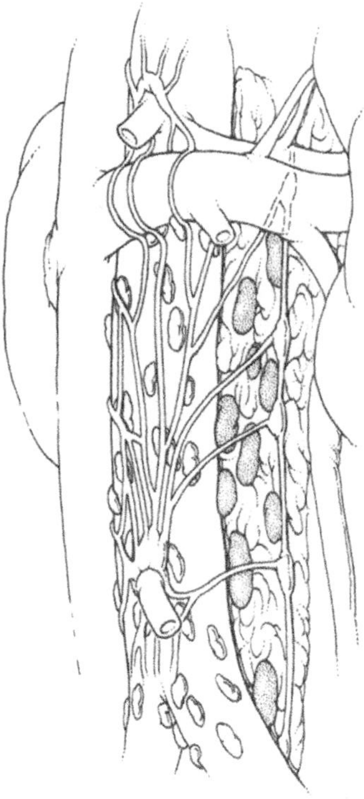

Figure 2. Left anterolateral view showing the relationships of the dorsal left sympathetic chain to the aorta. The postganglionic branches of L-1 through L-4 course anterior to the para-aortic nodes in the sulcus between the aorta and anterior spinous ligaments. A complete dissection requires removal of these nodes (stippled-shaded) as well as the more apparent set of nodes anterior to the aorta (not shaded).

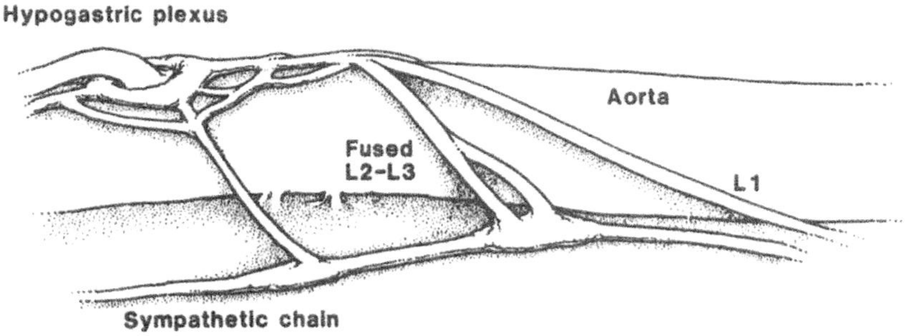

Figure 3. A left-sided view of the left para-aortic sympathetic chain and postganglionic fibers arising from ganglia of L-2 and L-3, which are often close to each other and sometimes seemingly fused. One can better appreciate the spatial relationships of the dorsal set of para-aortic nodes (stippled in Figures 2 and 3) to the nerve trunks after completion of NS-RPLND, as suggested by this figure.

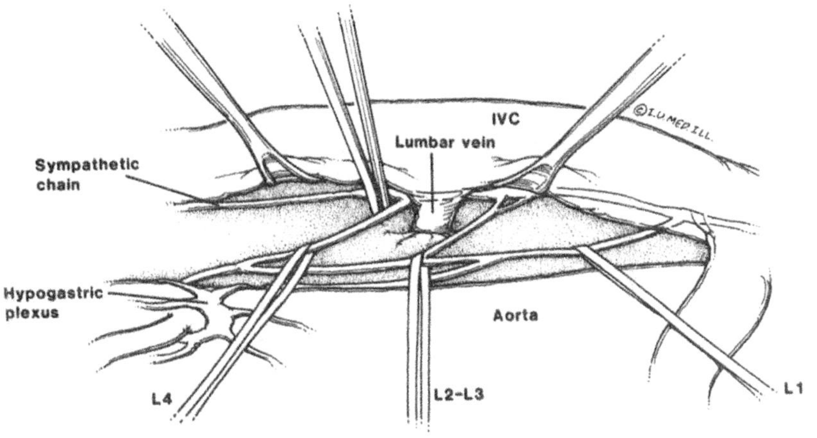

Figure 4. A view of the right sympathetic chain and its relationship to the vena cava, lumbar veins, and postganglionic nerve trunks that course medially across the interaortocaval space to join the pre-aortic hypogastric plexus. Division of the lumbar veins facilitates the exposure of the right sympathetic chain.

For a left-sided dissection, one of two approaches can be utilized. The root of the small bowel may be incised in the area of the duodenum with reflection of the duodenum cephalad and to the right, along with retraction of the mesentery of the left colon to the left and inferiorly (Figure 4). This exposes the upper interaortacaval zone and the upper left periaortic zone. The inferior mesenteric artery is left intact. Postganglionic sympathetic fibers are identified in the left periaortic zone distally, near the area of the inferior mesenteric artery. They are then dissected proximally in a prospective fashion, followed by retroperitoneal lymphadenectomy using the templates for left-sided dissection determined by previous mapping studies. The lower portion of the left periaortic zone is subsequently dissected after the sigmoid colon is flipped medially. This maneuver is also necessary to remove the remaining left internal spermatic vein.

An alternate approach is to mobilize the entire left colon medially as is done for radical nephrectomy, to identify the left-sided sympathetic fibers distally in the area of the bifurcation of the aorta, and to trace these fibers proximally to the sympathetic chain. After dissection of these fibers prospectively, standard lymphadenectomy is carried out as dictated by the template for left-sided dissection.

It should be emphasized that a complete en-bloc lymphadenectomy is performed as in full bilateral dissection. The only caveat is that the en bloc dissection is carried out after the prospective dissection of sympathetic fibers. Additionally, lumbar arteries and veins are divided only as needed and are not divided on a routine basis, as is done for full bilateral post-chemotherapy lymphadenectomy.

Our initial experience at Indiana University has been presented [2]. Currently we have a 2-year follow-up on 75 patients subjected to nerve-sparing retroperitoneal lymph node dissection [2]. All patients were clinical stage I; 14 cases were pathologic stage II. All 75 patients ejaculated postoperatively. Of the 14 pathologic stage II cases, four have relapsed. One patient had a documented retroperitoneal recurrence, was given full-dose chemotherapy, and subsequently underwent postchemotherapy retroperitoneal lymph node dissection. The pathology from this procedure showed only necrosis.

All patients are currently without evidence of disease. Details concerning the fertility status of these patients will be the subject of a future report.

The above mentioned experience documents the advance nerve-sparing retroperitoneal lymphadenectomy has yielded in the reduction of morbidity in the treatment of nonseminomatous testis cancer. Because of the suspected 60% incidence of abnormal spermatogenesis in patients presenting with this disease prior to any other therapy, it is unclear whether or not these patients will have normal fertility [14]. Therefore, we are following closely the fertility status in these patients postoperatively. In distinction to postchemotherapy retroperitoneal lymph-node dissection, the perioperative morbidity of staging lymphadenectomy in low-stage testicular cancer is exceedingly low. The average hospital stay is less than 1 week, and perioperative complications are exceedingly rare [15]. With the development of a technique that seems to retain the efficacy of lymphadenectomy but spares the patient the major source of morbidity, the argument against lymphadenectomy and for surveillance must be re-examined. This reduction of the major source of morbidity, coupled with the data of Hoskins and others showing a relapse rate of greater than 30% at 4 years, argues strongly against surveillance. Additionally, it is now known that 4–8% of this greater than 30% of patients who relapse on surveillance protocols relapse beyond 2 years after orchiectomy [16]. This is in contrast to the unlikely event of a recurrence greater than 2 years after lymphadenectomy.

Nerve-sparing lymphadenectomy must now be considered the standard surgical treatment for low-stage nonseminomatous carcinoma of the testis. Additionally, greater facility with these nerve-sparing techniques is likely to allow the preservation of ejaculatory ability in selected patients undergoing postchemotherapy dissection. These nerve-sparing techniques, therefore, enable the modern urologic oncologist to preserve the efficacy of a time-tested operation, at the same time eliminating its major source of morbidity.

References

1. Williams SD, Stablein DM, Einhorn LH, et al.: Immediate adjuvant chemotherapy versus observation with treatment of relapse in pathological stage II testicular cancer. *N Engl J Med* 317:1433–1438, 1987.

2. Donohue JP, Foster RS, Gelel G, et al.: Preservation of ejaculation following nerve-sparing retroperitoneal lymphadenectomy. J Urol 144:287, 1990.
3. Donohue JP, et al. Correlation of CAT changes and histological findings in 80 patients having RPLND after chemotherapy for testis cancer. J Urol 137:1176, 1987.
4. Loehrer PJ, Williams SD, Clark SA, et al.: Teratoma following chemotherapy for non-seminomatous germ cell tumor (NSGCT): A clinicopathologic correlation. J Urol 135:1183, 1986.
5. Einhorn LH, Williams SD, Mandelbaum I, Donohue JP: Surgical resection in disseminated testicular cancer following chemotherapeutic cytoreduction. Cancer 48:904–908, 1981.
6. Einhorn LH, Donohue JP: Cis-diammine-dichloroplatinum, vinblastine and bleomycin combination chemotherapy in disseminated testicular cancer. Ann Int Med 87:293–298, 1977.
7. Donohue JP, Einhorn LH, Williams SD: Cytoreductive surgery for metastatic testis cancer: Considerations of timing and extent. J Urol 123:876–880, 1980.
8. Donohue JP, Rowland RG: The role of surgery in advanced testicular cancer. Cancer 54:2716–2721, 1984.
9. Loehrer PJ, Sledge GW, Einhorn LH: Heterogeneity among germ cell tumors of the testis. Semin Oncol 12:304–316, 1985.
10. Ulbright TM, Loehrer PJ, Roth LM, et al.: The development of non-germ cell malignancies within germ cell tumors: A clinicopathologic study of 11 cases. Cancer 54:1824–1833, 1984.
11. Donohue JP, Zachary JM, Maynard BR: Distribution of nodal metastases in non-seminomatous testis cancer. J Urol 128:315–320, 1982.
12. Donohue JP, Rowland RG, Bihrle R: Transabdominal retroperitoneal lymph node dissection. In: Skinner, DG and Leiskovsky, G (eds). *Diagnosis and Management of Genitourinary Cancer*. W.B. Saunders, Philadelphia, 1988, pp. 802–816.
13. Donohue JP, Rowland RG: Complications of retroperitoneal lymphadenectomy. J Urol 125:338, 1981.
14. Lange PH, Chang WY, Fraley EE: Fertility issues in the therapy of nonseminomatous testicular tumors. Urol Clin North Am 14:731–745, 1987.
15. Bihrle R, Donohue JP, Foster RS: Complications of retroperitoneal lymph node dissection. Urol Clin North Am 15:237–242, 1988.
16. Hoskins P, Dilly S, Easton D: Prognostic factors in stage I nonseminomatous germ cell testicular tumors managed by orchiectomy and surveillance: Implications for adjuvant chemotherapy. J Clin Oncol 4:1031–1036, 1986.

9. Neoadjuvant chemotherapy and partial cystectomy for invasive bladder cancer

Harry W. Herr and Howard I. Scher

Cure of invasive bladder cancer is possible only if all disease is eradicated. For the primary tumor this usually requires total cystectomy. In selected cases, complete excision can be accomplished by TUR [1] or partial cystectomy [2]. These methods have the advantage of bladder preservation.

At first presentation, only 5–10% of invasive tumors are amenable to partial cystectomy [2]. In appropriately selected patients, survival is not compromised. A review of 128 patients undergoing partial cystectomy between 1946 and 1983 at MSKCC showed survival comparable to radical cystectomy [3]. For Ta-T1 lesions survivals were 75% vs. 61%, for T2-T3a 68% vs. 31%, and for T3b tumors 30% vs. 15%.

Definitive local control by any method does not assure a cure since relapses are common. The 5-year survival ranges from 30% to an optimistic 70%. Most patients succumb to metastatic disease. To improve the prognosis for patients with invasive bladder cancer, effective systemic therapy is required.

M-VAC chemotherapy can induce significant responses in primary and metastatic bladder cancer and in some cases can effect cures [4]. For the primary bladder cancer, M-VAC alone is not adequate therapy, since we observed significant clinical (T) errors in evaluating the true pathologic (P) response to chemotherapy [5]. Patients require definitive surgery, usually total cystectomy. At the same time, patients (and physicians) are reluctant to categorically accept cystectomy when the post M-VAC evaluation shows no tumor or noninvasive tumor.

In our evolving experience with neoadjuvant M-VAC chemotherapy for invasive bladder cancers, patients achieving an endoscopic complete response (T0) were increasingly managed by partial cystectomy. Of the first 53 definitive surgical procedures reported after M-VAC, 18 (34%) had partial cystectomy vs. 35 who underwent total cystectomy [6]. The aim was to preserve the bladder where possible, to document the pathologic response to M-VAC, and to surgically salvage patients who had microscopic infiltrating cancer undetected clinically. Further, we noted many tumors that initially would have required total cystectomy were downstaged to such an extent that partial cystectomy became technically feasible.

Lepor, H. and Lawson R.K., (eds.), Therapy for Genitourinary Cancer. *ISBN 0-7923-1412-3.*

How well do such patients fare? This is a preliminary report of our ongoing experience with neoadjuvant M-VAC and partial cystectomy for primary operable invasive bladder cancer.

Patients

Between July 1984 and July 1989, 32 patients with T2-T4a bladder cancers underwent a partial cystectomy after receiving a median of four (range 2–5) cycles of M-VAC. The follow-up after surgery was 19.5 months (range 6–60 months). During the same time period, 65 other patients had total cystectomy.

The selection of patients for segmental resection included clinically complete and significant partial responders to M-VAC. Such a response was documented by bimanual palpation and a repeat TUR after M-VAC. The area of the bladder involved with scar or residual neoplasm was judged feasible for a partial cystectomy with at least a 2-cm full-thickness bladder margin. Such patients had mobile bladders of adequate capacity and no palpable mass. CT scans were used to evaluate the response, but CT results did not deter a partial cystectomy if the endoscopic findings were favorable.

Prior multifocal disease and/or base locations were not considered contraindications if complete responses were documented in all or enough sites. In fact, partial cystectomy was done in all patients who showed sufficient tumor response to permit total excision of all areas of known invasive disease, consistent with restoration of a functional bladder. We realize the indications for partial cystectomy clearly have been extended in this group of patients.

Results

Of the 32 patients, only four were considered ideal candidates for partial cystectomy before M-VAC. The other 28 became amenable for segmental excision as a result of M-VAC. Most patients had solitary muscle-invasive cancers (average size, 4 × 4 cm) involving the base, lateral, or posterior walls of the bladder, and 10 (31%) had associated carcinoma in situ (Tis). In order to obtain the necessary margin, resection of the intramural ureter and ureteral reimplantation was required in seven patients, and liberal resection of the bladder neck and prostatic tissue in another six.

A typical case is shown in Figure 1. In January 1988 the patient presented with a T3a tumor involving the left ureteral orifice and diffuse basilar Tis. After two cycles of M-VAC, only atypical mucosa remained in the area of the invasive tumor. After two additional cycles, there was no endoscopic evidence of disease. In June 1988 a partial cystectomy, including the left ureteral orifice, was performed. No tumor (P0) was found in the specimen.

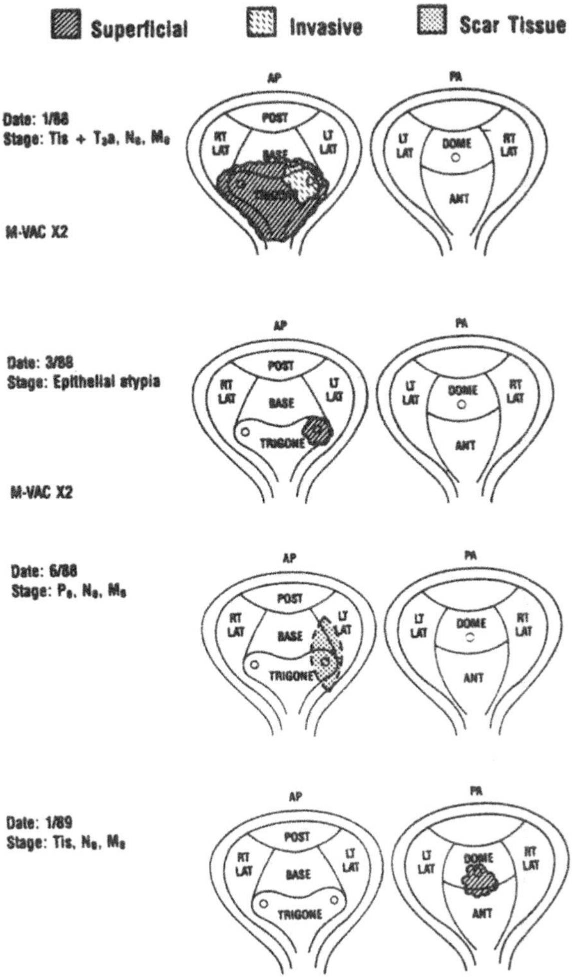

Figure 1. Clinical (+) and pathologic (p) response of an invasive (T3) bladder cancer to chemotherapy and partial cystectomy.

In January 1989, a patch of Tis was resected at the dome. There was no tumor involving the base. The patient received a 6-week course of intravesical BCG and remains tumor free with normal bladder function in January 1990, 2 years after his original diagnosis.

Table 1 shows the relation of the post M-VAC clinical (T) and pathologic (P) stages to the initial T stage. Seventy-two percent of the patients had either P0 (50%) or <P2 (22%) surgically. The overall accuracy of a TUR in predicting a complete pathologic response to M-VAC was 84% (16/19). The clinical accuracy in defining residual muscle-infiltrating disease was 97%. Only one patient with a T3a tumor believed T0 after M-VAC had P2+ disease at surgery.

Table 1. Relation of post M-VAC clinical (T) stage and pathologic (P) stage to initial T stage

		Post M-VAC T Stage			Post M-VAC P Stage		
Initial T Stage	No. Pts	TO	<T2	>T2	PO	<P2	>P2
T2	(7)	4 (57%)	—	3 (43%)	3 (43%)	1 (14%)	3 (43%)
T3a	(20)	12 (60%)	4 (20%)	4 (20%)	11 (55%)	4 (20%)	5 (25%)
T3b	(4)	3 (75%)	—	1 (25%)	2 (50%)	1 (25%)	1 (25%)
T4	(1)	—	1	—	—	1	—
Totals	32	19 (59%)	5 (16%)	8 (25%)	16 (50%)	7 (22%)	9 (28%)

Table 2. Relation of relapse pattern to pathologic response

		Relapse Pattern		No.	
PR	No. Pts	Bladder[a]	Systemic±	Bladder[b]	Relapse
PO	16	4	2		10
<P2	7	2	2		3
>P2	9	—	4		5
Totals	32	6 (19%)	8 (25%)		18 (56%)

[a] ALL Tis.
[b] 1T1, 3T2+

Table 3. Treatment outcome relative to pathologic response to M-VAC

			Outcome		
Post M-VAC P Stage	No. Pts.	Patient NED	AWD	DOD	DOC
P0	16	14 (88%)	—	1	1
<P2	7	5 (71%)	1	1	—
>P2	9	5 (56%)	2	2	—
Totals	32	24 (75%)	3	4	1

Table 2 shows relapses relative to the pathologic response to M-VAC. Most relapses (56%) are systemic, probably present at the time of diagnosis and resistant to chemotherapy. All relapses in the bladder alone (19%), to date, have been in situ carcinoma and all responded, at least in the short term, to BCG.

Table 3 shows the treatment outcome relative to the pathologic response to M-VAC. Of the 32 patients, 24 (75%) are disease free with functioning bladders over a median of 19 months. Disease-free survival is clearly better in patients achieving a complete (88%) or partial (71%) pathologic response.

Discussion

The present results are encouraging. M-VAC chemotherapy and extended partial cystectomy has achieved local control of the primary invasive bladder cancer and has preserved the bladder in some patients. Such patients are highly selected and follow-up is short. Treatment outcome results from a combination of multiple TURs, M-VAC chemotherapy, and partial cystectomy. There is no doubt that M-VAC has downstaged some tumors to permit partial excision and that such surgery has favorably consolidated the response to chemotherapy.

As long as the bladder remains, such patients are at risk to develop new invasive tumors. Will these occur at the same site as the original tumor or in other areas? Are patients with carcinoma in situ at higher risk for new invasive disease? Will M-VAC and surgery jeopardize the construction of a neobladder in the event that cystectomy becomes necessary for relapse? Much longer follow-up and more experience are needed before neoadjuvant chemotherapy and partial cystectomy can be considered a rational and safe option for selected patients with invasive bladder cancers.

References

1. Herr HW: Conservative management of muscle-infiltrating bladder cancer. J Urol 138:1162, 1987.
2. Whitmore WF: Management of invasive neoplasms. Semin Urol 1:4, 1983.
3. Whitmore WF: Personal communication.
4. Sternberg CN, Yagoda A, Scher HI, et al.: M-VAC (methotrexate, vinblastine, doxorubicin and cisplatin) for advanced transitional cell carcinoma of the urothelium. J Urol 139:461, 1988.
5. Scher HI, Herr HW, Yagoda A, et al.: Neoadjuvant M-VAC effect on the primary bladder lesion. J Urol 139:470, 1988.
6. Scher HI, Herr HW, Sternberg C, et al.: Neoadjuvant chemotherapy for invasive bladder cancer: Experience with the M-VAC regimen. Br J Urol 64:250, 1989.

10. Tumor necrosis factor and chemotherapeutic drugs targeted at DNA topoisomerase II for the treatment of genitourinary malignancies

Richard B. Alexander

Tumor necrosis factor (TNF) was first described in 1975 [1] as a soluble factor appearing in the serum of mice treated with BCG and endotoxin. This factor received its name because it caused the hemorrhagic necrosis of a transplantable sarcoma in mice. Subsequently, TNF was found to be a protein secreted by activated macrophages and was described in virtually all vertebrate animals, including humans. TNF was purified and the gene for human TNF was cloned and expressed in bacteria, making available large quantities of purified recombinant human TNF (rTNF) [2–4].

The mechanism of TNF's tumor necrosing activity remains unknown, although a tremendous amount of information regarding TNF's many activities has been learned. When rTNF became available, clinical trials of this material in patients with cancer were begun. While the final assessment of rTNF's antitumor efficacy in patients must await the conclusion of phase II trials, preliminary observations in phase I clinical trials of systemically administered rTNF as a single agent in the treatment of advanced human cancers have been disappointing (reviewed in [5]). TNF has substantial toxicity in these human trials, which has limited the dose that can be safely administered to patients.

However, while rTNF as a single agent appears likely to be of limited clinical usefulness in human cancers, this factor has many interesting and potentially useful anticancer interactions with other cytokines and chemotherapeutic agents. For example, rTNF has demonstrated synergistic antitumor effects with the interferons and with interleukin-2 (IL-2) [6–10]. TNF also has interactions with chemotherapeutic drugs. TNF and dactinomycin have synergistic antitumor effects in murine models, and this association is exploited in the TNF bioassay [11]. Recently, it was recognized that synergistic antitumor effects similar to that seen with rTNF and dactinomycin are also observed when rTNF is combined with a class of chemotherapeutic drugs, of which dactinomycin is a member. These agents are those targeted at the enzyme DNA topoisomerase II [12,13] and include some of the most frequently used drugs in human cancers.

This chapter will review the combination of rTNF and topoisomerase II-targeted drugs, particularly with regard to urologic malignancies. The com-

Lepor, H. and Lawson R.K., (eds.), Therapy for Genitourinary Cancer. *ISBN 0-7923-1412-3.*

bination of these two diverse agents has interesting biologic effects, which may provide insight into how both TNF and topoisomerase II-targeted drugs are lethal to cells, and may suggest new strategies for the therapy of human cancers.

TNF brief review

TNF was first described in 1975 as a soluble factor appearing in the serum of mice treated with BCG and bacterial endotoxin [1]. The serum from such mice contained a factor that, when injected intravenously (i.v.), caused the hemorrhagic necrosis of a transplantable murine sarcoma called Meth A. TNF was subsequently found to have a large number of functions, in addition to this tumor necrosing activity. TNF is a protein of molecular weight 17,000 that is secreted by activated macrophages and is best classified as a cytokine, one of a large group of soluble factors secreted by cells of the immune system. TNF's function as a regulator of the immune system is also suggested by the finding that the gene for TNF is closely linked to the major histocompatibility complex (MHC), which codes for the expression of cell-surface recognition molecules of critical importance to the immune system. As with other cytokines, TNF's many effects are mediated by high-affinity receptors [8], and such receptors have been found on virtually all nucleated cells. TNF has effects on vascular endothelium [14,15], lymphocytes, neutrophils [16], and other reticuloendothelial cells and appears to be involved in the pathophysiology of septic shock [17,18], cachexia [19], and chronic granulomatous diseases, such as tuberculosis [20]. The physiology of TNF is quite complex and the subject of intense study. Thus TNF, like other biological response modifiers, has numerous activities that might be beneficial or harmful when used as a therapeutic agent.

TNF and anticancer effects

The initial impetus for the study of TNF was the observation of hemorrhagic necrosis in some experimental murine tumors caused by a single i.v. injection of TNF. While hemorrhagic necrosis was not observed in all tumors in the murine models, TNF alone was not only capable of causing hemorrhagic necrosis and regression of established tumor, but could also cure a substantial proportion of the animals [21]. Studies of the mechanism of TNF's tumor-necrosing activity can be summarized as follows: 1) hemorrhagic necrosis occurs over a few hours after a single i.v. bolus of TNF; 2) hemorrhagic necrosis occurs only in larger tumors (>5 mm diameter), both in subcutaneous and organ-based sites [22]; 3) no effects on small experimental metastatic tumors have been observed [22]; 4) hemorrhagic necrosis is not just a consequence of the tumors being transplanted, because

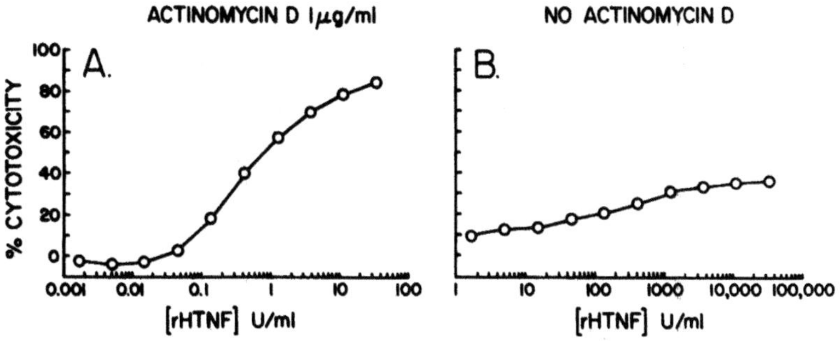

Figure 1. Comparison of L929 cytotoxicity from recombinant human TNF (rHTNF, Cetus, specific activity 2 × 10^7 U/mg protein) in the presence (panel A) or absence (panel B) of dactinomycin (actinomycin D). Note different scale of x axes and relative lack of cytotoxic effect of rTNF alone in the absence of dactinomycin.

autochthonous newly induced tumors in mice undergo hemorrhagic necrosis following TNF injection [23]; and 5) cure of tumors following hemorrhagic necrosis from TNF requires an intact host cellular immune system [24,25].

In addition to TNF's activity against tumors in vivo, it was recognized quite early that TNF had direct cytotoxic effects on some tumor cells in vitro. The anticancer specificity of TNF in vitro appeared to be preserved, as TNF did not have cytotoxic effects on normal cells and, in fact, could act as a growth factor for some normal cells in culture [26]. The cytotoxic activity of TNF in vitro against the murine fibrosarcoma L929 is the basis of the TNF bioassay. The assay is performed by exposing monolayers of L929 cells in 96-well plates to various concentrations of TNF, generally for 18–24 hours. At the end of the incubation period, the cells are stained and treated monolayers are compared to control monolayers photometrically (the intensity of staining is proportional to the number of cells). The percent cytotoxicity is the fraction of cells in treated monolayers compared to control monolayers. Another early observation about TNF's antitumor activity in this assay was that the cytotoxic effect of TNF on the cells was greatly increased in the presence of dactinomycin, as shown in Figure 1. The addition of this drug to the TNF bioassay is now standard.

While TNF has direct cytotoxic activity on tumor cells in vitro, it appears that hemorrhagic necrosis seen in vivo is not related to the direct cytotoxic effect on tumor cells seen in vitro. The best evidence for this conclusion is that Meth A and a variety of other chemically induced murine sarcomas that readily demonstrate hemorrhagic necrosis in vivo from i.v. TNF are completely resistant to TNF in vitro (R.B. Alexander, unpublished observations). Thus mechanisms other than direct cytotoxicity are believed responsible for the hemorrhagic necrosis of tumors observed in vivo. TNF's effects on vasculature [14,15] and TNF's immunomodulating properties are possible mechanisms of hemorrhagic necrosis.

TNF and dactinomycin

The combination of TNF and dactinomycin greatly increases the cytotoxicity observed against L929 cells in vitro compared to TNF alone (see Figure 1). The addition of dactinomycin decreases the time of incubation needed for maximum cytotoxicity to be observed. In the absence of dactinomycin, TNF's direct antiproliferative effect on L929 cells requires prolonged incubation (3–5 days), but in the presence of 1µg/ml dactinomycin, this time is shortened to less than 24 hours [11]. Dactinomycin has numerous effects on cells but is a potent inhibitor of protein synthesis and mRNA transcription. It was thus postulated that protein synthesis inhibition prevented some type of repair process induced by TNF, and this was responsible for the synergistic cytotoxicity of the combination [27].

Several subtleties of the interaction of TNF and dactinomycin deserve further scrutiny. The cytotoxic effect of TNF is calculated by comparing TNF-treated cells with control cells not exposed to TNF. When dactinomycin is added to the medium, both control cells and TNF-treated cells are exposed to dactinomycin, and thus the antiproliferative effect of dactinomycin alone is cancelled out. What fraction of cytotoxicity observed in L929 cells in vitro from TNF plus dactinomycin might be due to dactinomycin alone? In fact, we were surprised to observe that in an 18-hour assay in the absence of dactinomycin, rTNF had no cytotoxicity to L929 cells at concentrations of rTNF that caused maximum cytotoxicity in the presence of dactinomycin. By examining the effect of each agent alone and in combination with the control cells exposed to medium alone, as shown in Figure 2, it was clear that dactinomycin had dose-dependent cytotoxicity to L929 cells and that this cytotoxicity was enhanced in the presence of rTNF at concentrations of rTNF that alone had no detectable effect on the cells at 18 hours [12]. Thus, when compared to medium alone, dactinomycin had significant cytotoxicity to L929 cells, and this cytotoxicity was enhanced by the addition of rTNF.

Topoisomerase II

In addition to inhibiting protein synthesis, dactinomycin has numerous other effects on cells. Recently, dactinomycin has been shown to interact with the nuclear enzyme DNA topoisomerase II and to inhibit part of the function of this enzyme [28]. Topoisomerases are enzymes that catalyze the winding and unwinding of DNA [reviewed in references 29 and 30]. There are two topoisomerases in mammalian cells — topoisomerase I and II — which have enzymatic activity for single- and double-stranded DNA, respectively. These enzymes are of critical importance to the cell and are involved in the regulation of DNA transcription and translation. Topoisomerases are a major component of the nuclear matrix, a scaffold-like structure to which DNA is attached in the nucleus, and topoisomerases also form the central core of chromosomes [31].

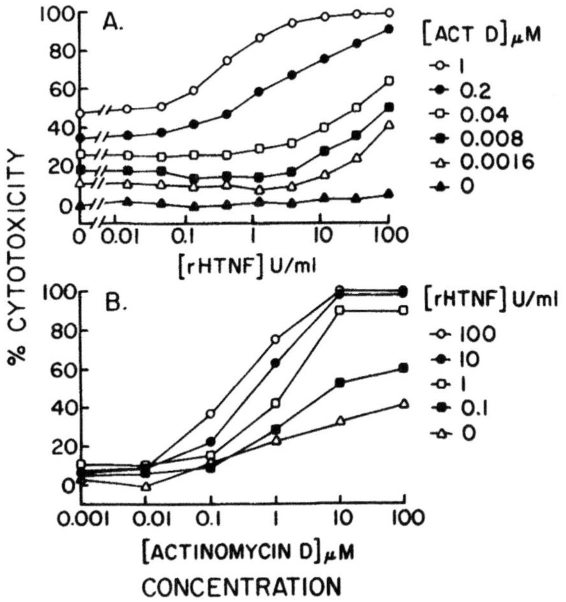

Figure 2. Effect of recombinant human TNF (rHTNF, Cetus, specific activity 2 × 10^7 U/mg protein) and dactinomycin (actinomycin D) on L929 cells. Note in panel A that cytotoxicity is shown as a function of rHTNF concentration, which in the absence of dactinomycin rHTNF had no cytotoxic effect. In panel B, similar data from a different experiment are shown with cytotoxicity as a function of the dactinomycin concentration. Note that dactinomycin clearly has a dose-dependent cytotoxic effect on the cells that is increased in the presence of rHTNF at various fixed concentrations, as shown. From R.B. Alexander et al. [12], reproduced with permission.

The function of topoisomerase II is depicted schematically in Figure 3. The enzyme functions by covalently binding to double-stranded DNA, breaking the strand, passing a different strand through the break, and then religating the strand and detaching. This strand-passing activity is crucial to the cell during transcription of mRNA, and also during DNA synthesis and mitosis, when daughter strands of DNA must be packaged into separate chromosomes. Drugs targeted at topoisomerase II, such as dactinomycin, interfere with the strand-passing activity of the enzyme. The enzyme attaches to DNA and nicks the strand but cannot progress past this point. This results in DNA breaks with the enzyme covalently attached, and this form of DNA damage is felt to be the lesion that is lethal to the cell. A variety of agents have been found to have topoisomerase II-targeted activity, and this includes some of the most widely used chemotherapeutic agents in human cancers. A partial listing of these drugs is shown in Table 1. These drugs have different physical properties; some, such as dactinomycin and doxorubicin, intercalate DNA, while others, such as etoposide (VP-16), do not bind to DNA.

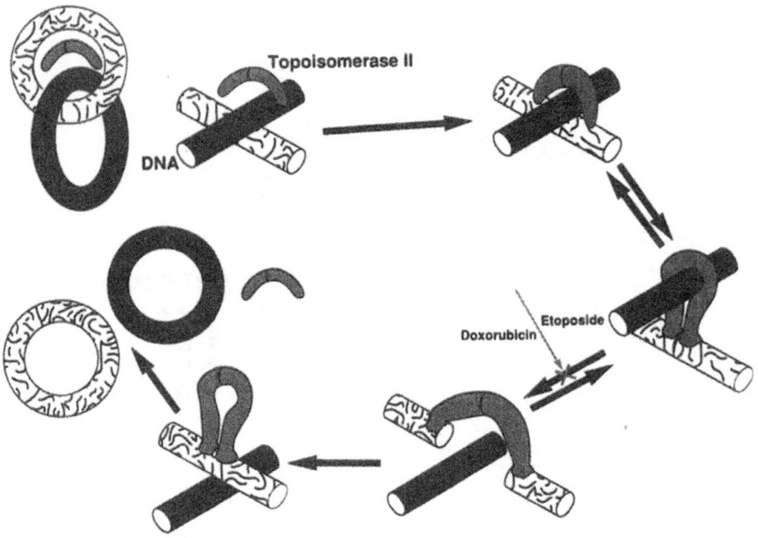

Figure 3. Schematic representation of the function of DNA topoisomerase II. Concatenated rings of double-stranded DNA are shown. The enzyme covalently attaches to one strand of DNA, breaks the strand, passes the other strand through, religates the DNA strand, and detaches. Drugs such as etoposide and doxorubicin block the function of the enzyme at the point shown. This results in the accumulation of DNA breaks covalently attached to topoisomerase. Figure (with modifications) courtesy of Kurt W. Kohn.

Table 1. Chemotherapeutic agents targeted at DNA topoisomerase II

Dactinomycin (actinomycin D)
Doxorubicin (adriamycin)
Etoposide (VP-16)
Teniposide (VM-26)
mAMSA (Amsacrine)

TNF and topoisomerase II-targeted drugs in vitro

We asked if the enhancement of L929 cytotoxicity that occurs when TNF and dactinomycin are combined could be related to dactinomycin's effect on topoisomerase II. One way to examine this question was to combine TNF with other topoisomerase II-targeted drugs in the L929 assay. In fact, TNF demonstrated cytotoxic synergy in the L929 assay with all of the topoisomerase II-targeted drugs, but not with other DNA-damaging drugs not targeted at topoisomerase II [12], as shown in Figure 4. This suggests that TNF's enhancement of cytotoxicity is in some way related to the topoisomerase II-inhibiting activity of these drugs.

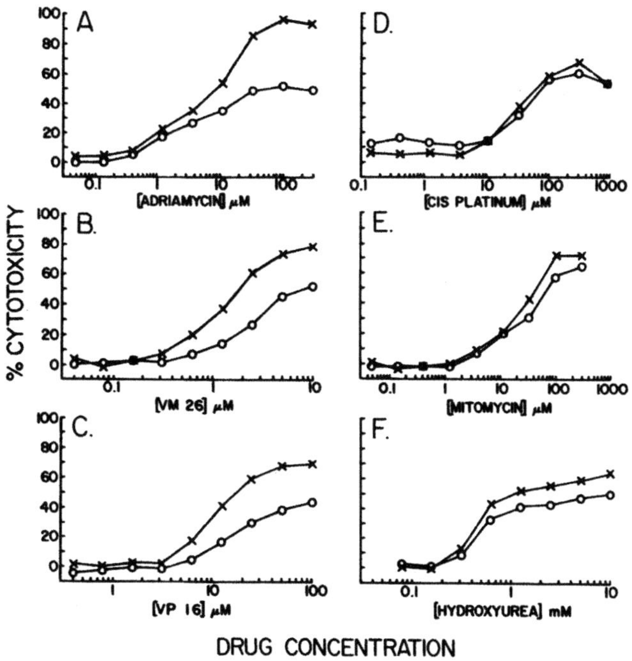

Figure 4. Effect of rTNF and various drugs on L929 cells. L929 cells were exposed to various drugs in the absence (–O–) or presence (–×–) of recombinant human TNF (rHTNF, Cetus, specific activity 2 × 10^7 U/mg protein), 100 U/ml. Note that rHTNF increases the cytotoxic effect of doxorubicin (adriamycin), teniposide (VM-26), and etoposide (VP-16), all of which are targeted at DNA topoisomerase II, but not cisplatin, mitomycin C, or hydroxyurea, none of which interact with topoisomerase II. Modified from R.B. Alexander et al. [12]. Reproduced with permission.

Similar findings have been reported in other in vitro tumor models. Freuhauf et al. demonstrated synergistic cytotoxicity against the human prostatic cancer cell line LNCaP when TNF and doxorubicin were combined [32]. The murine bladder tumor line MBT-2 demonstrated enhanced cytotoxicity in the presence of TNF and topoisomerase II-targeted agents [13,33]. TNF has also been shown to enhance the cytotoxic effect of dactinomycin and doxorubicin in human squamous carcinoma cell lines, whereas TNF did not enhance the cytotoxicity of cisplatin, methotrexate, or fluorouracil against the same cell lines [34].

Clearly, not all tumor cell lines are sensitive to TNF in vitro, even those that express high-affinity receptors for TNF. It does not appear that topoisomerase-targeted agents can convert a resistant cell to become sensitive. For example, Giaconne et al. found that several human lung-cancer cell lines were resistant to TNF, although several expressed TNF receptors; neither doxorubicin nor etoposide could convert any of these resistant lines to TNF sensitivity [35].

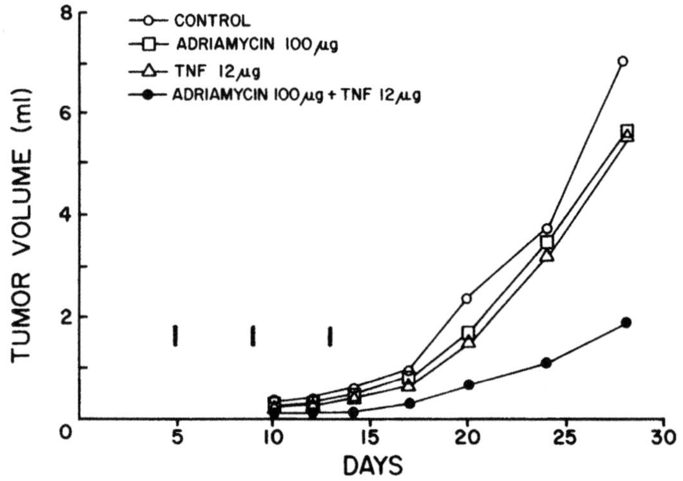

Figure 5. Growth curve of subcutaneous MBT-2 bladder tumor in C3H/He mice. Animals received 25-mg trocar pieces of MBT-2 tumor on day 0 followed by rTNF or doxorubicin (adriamycin) intraperitoneally for 3 doses (vertical lines). Only the combination of rTNF plus doxorubicin had an antitumor effect; rTNF or doxorubicin alone were indistinguishable from controls.

TNF and topoisomerase II-targeted drugs in vivo

While synergistic cytotoxicity in vitro is interesting, findings derived from cells in culture may bear little resemblance to those from animal studies. Nevertheless, numerous studies have shown that the antitumor relationship of the combination of TNF and the topoisomerase II-targeted drugs also occurs in vivo. The MBT-2 murine bladder tumor line growing in the subcutaneous space in C3H/He mice demonstrated sensitivity to the combination of TNF and etoposide, and TNF and dactinomycin, when each agent alone had no effect [13]. A similar finding for doxorubicin (adriamycin) and rTNF is shown in Figure 5. In these studies, rTNF and chemotherapy were administered intraperitoneally; similar findings have been reported for intratumoral rTNF and systemic etoposide in MBT-2 [36]. In other mouse tumor models, rTNF and doxorubicin had a better antitumor effect than either agent alone in the murine sarcoma MCA 106 [37], and also in a model of solitary liver sarcoma in the rat [38].

Human tumor cell lines grown in athymic nu/nu (nude) mice provide the opportunity to examine these relationships using human tumors in an in vivo setting, although the relevance to human cancer is limited. Das et al. [39] demonstrated synergism between rTNF and etoposide in human transitional cell carcinoma grown beneath the renal capsule in nude mice. Similar findings for human renal cell carcinoma in nude mice have been reported [40,41]. The toxicity of TNF and topoisomerase-targeted drugs in the limited animal trials available has been, for the most part, acceptable, although significant toxicity from the combination therapy has been described [37]. Thus, the cytotoxic synergy between TNF and topoisomerase-targeted drugs occurs both in vitro and in vivo.

Mechanism of synergistic antitumor effects

The mechanism of TNF and topoisomerase-targeted drug synergy is unknown. However, several recent observations about the interaction are germane to this discussion. First, the combination of TNF and topoisomerase II-targeted drugs causes an increase in cell death and not just an arrest of proliferation. L929 cells growing exponentially double every 24 hours. The incubation period of L929 cells in the TNF assay with dactinomycin is 18 hours, less than one doubling time. Note in Figures 1 and 4 that exposure to topoisomerase-targeted drugs and rTNF can cause greater than 90% cell destruction in less than one doubling time. A simple arrest of proliferation would yield 50% cytotoxicity compared to untreated cells in one doubling time. In fact, a careful examination of Figures 2 and 4 shows that continuous exposure of L929 cells to chemotherapeutic drugs for 18 hours yields a maximum cytotoxicity of 40–60%, as would be expected for cells unable to divide for one doubling time. It is only with the addition of rTNF that an increase in cell death occurs with cytotoxicity of 80–90% at 18 hours. This point is further illustrated by the appearance of the cells after the 18-hour incubation, as shown in Figure 6. Note that cells exposed to etoposide only remain intact (although spread out and with large uncondensed nuclei), but that the addition of rTNF to etoposide causes the destruction of most of the cells in the monolayer.

This argument is further supported by our recent observation using cell-cycle analysis that L929 cells exposed to topoisomerase II-targeted drugs accumulate in G_2M, the phase of the cell cycle where DNA has duplicated but the cell has not yet divided (unpublished observations). The cells are still viable in this state after the 18-hour incubation. This is consistent with the inhibition of topoisomerase II, leading to an inability of the cells to divide. Exposure to rTNF alone is indistinguishable from control cells exposed to medium only. However, exposure to TNF and topoisomerase II-targeted drugs leads to rapid cell death, such that virtually no viable cells remain at 18 hours. Thus, the combination of rTNF and topoisomerase II-targeted drugs results in an increase in cell death.

Second, it is well known that TNF causes fragmentation of target cell DNA into 200 base-pair multimers [42], typically seen in cells undergoing programmed cell death or apoptosis [43]. This internucleosomal DNA fragmentation is by no means specific for TNF-mediated cell death and

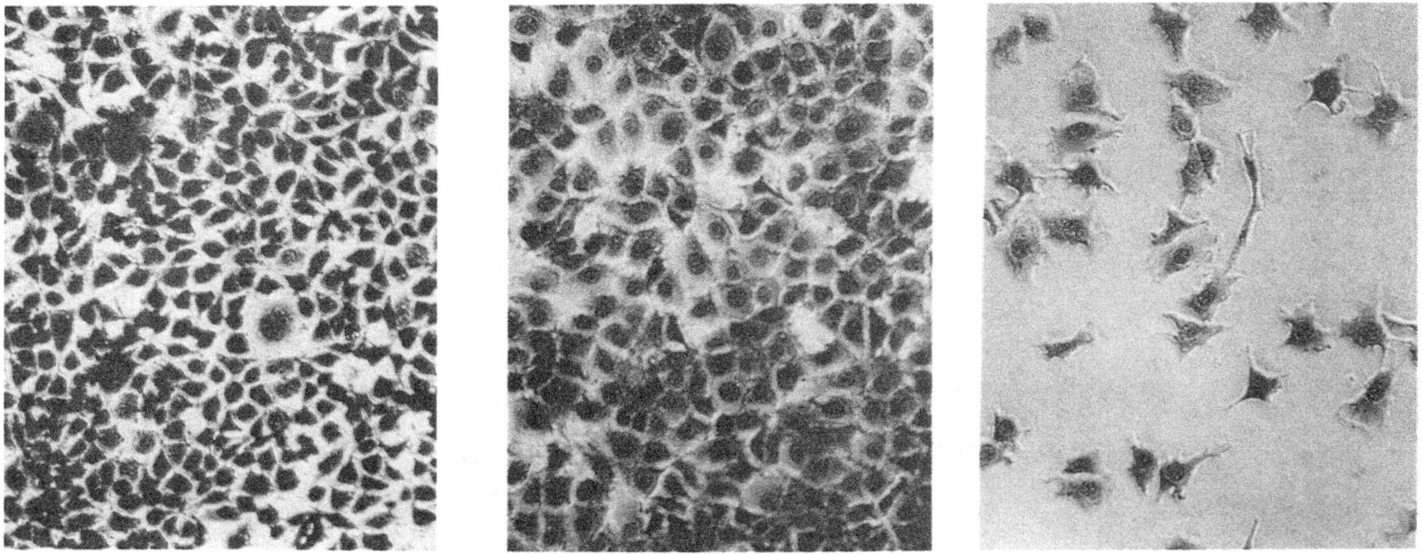

Figure 6. Histological appearance of L929 monolayers exposed to etoposide and rTNF. Exponentially growing L929 cells were exposed for 18 hours to medium only (left panel), etoposide 100 μM (center panel), or etoposide 100 μM plus rTNF 100 U/ml (right panel). Note that cells exposed to etoposide only show enlarged and uncondensed nuclei, and are more spread out, but remain intact. Cells exposed to the combination of etoposide and rTNF have mostly been destroyed, have detached from the monolayer, and are represented by the small residual bodies out of the plane of focus. Cells exposed to rTNF alone were indistinguishable from controls.

is probably a manifestation of cell death from a variety of causes [44]. However, as shown by Kyprianou et al. [45], this DNA fragmentation is accelerated by the addition of topoisomerase II-targeted drugs to TNF in vitro. This further supports the conclusion that TNF and these drugs cause an increase in cell death.

Third, Utsugi et al. [46] have recently shown that L929 cells manifest a rapid but brief increase in extractable topoisomerase activity following TNF exposure. They also confirmed our previous observation that synergy in vitro is observed only if topoisomerase-targeted drug exposure precedes or is coincident with exposure to TNF. Synergy is not observed if TNF exposure precedes topoisomerase-targeted drug exposure [12,46]. These findings are consistent with a model whereby the amount of lethal DNA damage caused by the topoisomerase-targeted drugs is increased by a transient rise in topoisomerase activity caused by TNF. The increase in cell death would then follow from this increased DNA damage. Alternately TNF may in some way increase programmed cell death, a metabolically active process undoubtedly requiring controlling factors and signals.

TNF and topoisomerase-targeted drugs in human cancer

The combination of rTNF and topoisomerase-targeted drugs has entered clinical trials in patients with advanced cancer. Preliminary reports of some of these trials using rTNF in combination with doxorubicin or etoposide are available [47–50]. These are phase I trials designed only to measure toxicity; no antitumor responses have been reported in a variety of advanced cancers. Recombinant TNF plus etoposide or rTNF plus doxorubicin have been administered by various schedules of continuous infusion or intravenous bolus. Toxicity in these preliminary trials has been acceptable and similar to that seen with rTNF alone, mainly fever, rigors, and hypotension. Thrombocytopenia and other hematologic toxicities have also been observed. It appears that the maximum tolerated dose of rTNF may be substantially lower when combined with chemotherapy. However, these preliminary data involve different dose schedules, and in some trials the maximum tolerated dose has not been reached. The assessment of efficacy of rTNF and topoisomerase-targeted drugs in human cancer will require the completion of trials to define toxicity and maximum tolerated dose, as well as phase II trials in a variety of cancers.

Future prospects

The major limitation to the use of rTNF in patients appears to be toxicity. The dose of rTNF that humans can tolerate is less than that which is needed to cause hemorrhagic necrosis in murine tumors [5]. Thus rTNF, as a single agent administered systemically, appears to have little chance of making a major impact upon human cancer. Strategies such as the combination of rTNF with chemotherapeutic drugs, which may exploit the antitumor effects of TNF at doses that can be administered to patients, should continue to be explored. In addition to systemic therapy, however, other routes of administration may be useful. Significant antitumor activity has been clearly shown when rTNF is injected directly into human cancers [5,51]. The regression of human tumors seen with intralesional rTNF suggests that rTNF can be effective in human cancer, but only when present in a high concentration; the failure of systemic rTNF administration to cause tumor regressions in patients may be because such high concentrations cannot be achieved with systemic administration at tolerable doses.

In this regard, another method of administration causing high local concentrations of drugs is intravesical therapy. Intravesical chemotherapy with a variety of agents for superficial bladder cancer is well established. There is also some experience with intravesical rTNF. A preliminary trial of rTNF in cynomolgus monkeys showed no evidence of toxicity [52], and a trial in humans with superficial bladder cancer is in progress (M. Ernstoff, personal communication). Doxorubicin has well-known activity against superficial bladder cancer, and intravesical TNF plus doxorubicin is a logical combination that might be explored in that disease. Toxicity would likely be less with intravesical therapy compared to intravenous administration. Another route of administration that might be used is intraperitoneal injection for advanced intraperitoneal cancer, such as ovarian carcinoma [53].

Another potential area of interest is the use of tumor-infiltrating lymphocytes (TIL) transduced with the gene for human TNF, studies currently underway at the Surgery Branch of the National Cancer Institute. TIL are lymphocytes obtained from solid tumors that are expanded in vitro in IL-2 and reinfused into patients with advanced cancer. TIL can be transduced using retroviral vectors, and such transduced cells have been used to trace TIL in patients after injection [54,55]. TIL from human cancers have also been transduced with the gene for TNF, and such cells secrete large amounts of TNF (A. Kasid, manuscript in preparation). Since TIL traffic to and accumulate in tumor deposits in patients, it is hoped that high concentrations of TNF will be secreted into the substance of tumors, resulting in an antitumor effect. The addition of topoisomerase-targeted drugs to this regimen is another potential area for further study.

Summary

Recombinant TNF as a single agent for human cancer appears to be of limited value. However, rTNF has synergistic anticancer effects when combined with chemotherapeutic drugs targeted at DNA topoisomerase II. This effect of rTNF has been observed in several in vitro and in vivo tumor models, both in animal and human studies. The mechanism of this interaction appears to involve lesions to the DNA of tumor cells mediated by inhibition of DNA topoisomerase II. The combinations of rTNF plus doxorubicin and rTNF plus etoposide administered systemically are currently under evaluation by clinical trials in patients with advanced cancers. Determination of the efficacy of such combination therapy must await the completion of phase I and II trails. Other routes of administration that might increase the local concentration of rTNF and could be combined with topoisomerase II-targeted drugs include intravesical administration and the use of tumor-infiltrating lymphocytes.

Acknowledgment

The author is indebted to Donald S. Coffey for inspiration, support, and good advice.

References

1. Carswell EA, Old LJ, Kasel RL, Green S, Fiore N, Williamson B: An endotoxin-induced serum factor that causes necrosis of tumors. Proc Natl Acad Sci USA, 72:3666–3670, 1975.
2. Pennica D, Hayflick JS, Bringman TS, Palladino MA, Goeddel DV: Cloning and expression in Escherichia coli of the cDNA for murine tumor necrosis factor. Proc Natl Acad Sci USA, 82:6060–6064, 1985.
3. Wang AM, Creasey AA, Ladner MB, Lin LS, Strickler J, Van Arsdell JN, Yamamoto R, Mark DF: Molecular cloning of the complementary DNA for human tumor necrosis factor. Science 228:149–154, 1985.
4. Shirai T, Yamaguchi H, Ito H, Todd CW, Wallace RB: Cloning and expression in Escherichia coli of the gene for human tumour necrosis factor. Nature 313:803–806, 1985.
5. Alexander RB, Rosenberg SA: Tumor necrosis factor: Clinical applications. In: DeVita VT, Hellman S, Rosenberg SA (eds). *Biologic Therapy of Cancer: Principles and Practice.* J.B. Lippincott, Philadelphia, 1990.
6. McIntosh JK, Mulé JJ, Merino MJ, Rosenberg SA: Synergistic antitumor effects of immunotherapy with recombinant interleukin-2 and recombinant tumor necrosis factor-alpha. Cancer Res 48:4011–4017, 1988.
7. Stone-Wolff DS, Yip YK, Kelker HC, Le J, Henriksen-Destefano D, Rubin BY, Rinderknecht E, Aggarwal BB, Vilcěk J: Interrelationships of human interferon-gamma with lymphotoxin and monocyte cytotoxin. J Exp Med 159:828–843, 1984.
8. Aggarwal BB, Eessalu TE, Hass PE: Characterization of receptors for human tumour necrosis factor and their regulation by gamma-interferon. Nature 318:665–667, 1985.
9. Kavoussi LR, Ruesing RA, Hudson MA, Catalona WJ, Ratliff TL: Effect of tumor necrosis factor and interferon gamma on human renal carcinoma cell line growth. J Urol 142:875–878, 1989.
10. McIntosh JK, Mulé JJ, Krosnick JA, Rosenberg SA: Combination cytokine immunotherapy with tumor necrosis factor alpha, interleukin 2, and alpha-interferon and its synergistic antitumor effects in mice. Cancer Res 49:1408–1414, 1989.
11. Ruff MR, Gifford GE: Tumor necrosis factor. In: Pick E (ed). *Lymphokines*, Vol. 2. Academic Press, New York, 1981, pp. 235–271.
12. Alexander RB, Nelson WG, Coffey DS: Synergistic enhancement by tumor necrosis factor

of in vitro cytotoxicity from chemotherapeutic drugs targeted at DNA topoisomerase II. Cancer Res 47:2403–2406, 1987.

13. Alexander RB, Isaacs JT, Coffey DS: Tumor necrosis factor enhances the in vitro and in vivo efficacy of chemotherapeutic drugs targeted at DNA topoisomerase II in the treatment of murine bladder cancer. J Urol 138:427–429, 1987.
14. Bevilacqua MP, Pober JS, Majeau GR, Fiers W, Cortran RS, Gimbrone MA, Jr.: Recombinant tumor necrosis factor induces procoagulant activity in cultured human vascular endothelium: Characterization and comparison with the actions of interleukin 1. Proc Natl Acad Sci USA 83:4533–4537, 1986.
15. Stolpen AH, Guinan EC, Fiers W, Pober JS: Recombinant tumor necrosis factor and immune interferon act singly and in combination to reorganize human vascular endothelial cell monolayers. Am J Pathol 123:16–24, 1986.
16. Tennenberg SD, Solomkin JS: Activation of neutrophils by cachectin/tumor necrosis factor: Priming of N-formyl-methionyl-leucyl-phenylalanine-induced oxidative responsiveness via receptor mobilization without degranulation. J Leuk Biol 47:217–223, 1990.
17. Beutler B, Milsark IW, Cerami AC: Passive immunization against cachectin/tumor necrosis factor protects mice from lethal effect of endotoxin. Science 229:869–871, 1985.
18. Michie HR, Manogue KR, Spriggs DR, Revhaug A, O'Dwyer S, Dinarello CA, Cerami A, Wolff SM, Wilmore DW: Detection of circulating tumor necrosis factor after endotoxin administration. N Engl J Med 318:1481–1486, 1988.
19. Levine B, Kalman J, Mayer L, Fillit HM, Packer M: Elevated circulating levels of tumor necrosis factor in severe chronic heat failure. N Engl J Med 323:236–241, 1990.
20. Rook GAW, Taverne J, Moreno C: The role of tumor necrosis factor in the pathogenesis of tuberculosis and leprosy and the relationship between tissue-damaging pathology and production of agalactosyl IgG. In: Bonavida B, Granger G (eds). *Tumor Necrosis Factor: Structure, Mechanism of Action, Role in Disease and Therapy*. Karger, Basel, 1990, pp. 168–176.
21. Creasey AA, Reynolds MT, Laird W: Cures and Partial regression of murine and human tumors by recombinant human tumor necrosis factor. Cancer Res 46:5687–5690, 1986.
22. Mulé JJ, Asher A, McIntosh J, Lafreniere R, Shiloni E, Lefor A, Reichert CM, Rosenberg SA: Antitumor effect of recombinant tumor necrosis factor-alpha against murine sarcomas at visceral sites: Tumor size influences the response to therapy. Cancer Immunol Immunother 26:202–208, 1988.
23. McIntosh JK, Mulé JJ, Travis WD, Rosenberg SA: Studies of effects of recombinant human tumor necrosis factor on autochthonous tumor and transplanted normal tissue in mice. Cancer Res 50:2463–2469, 1990.
24. Asher AL, Mulé JJ, Rosenberg SA: Recombinant human tumor necrosis factor mediates regression of a murine sarcoma in vivo via Lyt-2+ cells. Cancer Immunol Immunother 28:153–156, 1989.
25. Havell EA, Fiers W, North RJ: The antitumor function of tumor necrosis factor (TNF), I. Therapeutic action of TNF against an established murine sarcoma is indirect, immunologically dependent, and limited by severe toxicity. J Exp Med 167:1067–1085, 1988.
26. Sugarman BJ, Aggarwal BB, Hass PE, Figari IS, Palladino MA, Jr., Shepard HM: Recombinant human tumor necrosis factor-alpha: Effects on proliferation of normal and transformed cells in vitro. Science 230:943–945, 1985.
27. Ostrove JM, Gifford GE: Stimulation of RNA synthesis in L929 cells by rabbit tumor necrosis factor. Proc Soc Exp Biol Med 160:354–358, 1979.
28. Tewey KM, Rowe TC, Yang L, Halligan BD, Liu LF: Adriamycin-induced DNA damage mediated by mammalian DNA topoisomerase II. Science 226:466–468, 1984.
29. Liu LF: DNA topoisomerases — enzymes that catalyze the breaking and rejoining of DNA. CRC Crit Rev Biochem 15:1–24, 1983.
30. D'Arpa P, Liu LF: Topoisomerase-targeting antitumor drugs. Biochim Biophys Acta 989: 163–177, 1989.

31. Pienta KJ, Partin AW, Coffey DS: Cancer as a disease of DNA organization and dynamic cell structure. Cancer Res 49:2525–2532, 1989.
32. Fruehauf JP, Myers CE, Sinha BK: Synergistic activity of suramin with tumor necrosis factor alpha and doxorubicin on human prostate cancer cell lines. J Natl Cancer Inst 82:1206–1209, 1990.
33. Bahnson RR, Ratliff TL: In vitro and in vivo anti-tumor activity of recombinant mouse tumor necrosis factor (TNF) in a mouse bladder tumor (MBT-2). J Urol 144:172–175, 1990.
34. Gapany M, Dawson DE, Schriever C, Burgess R, Gipple JR, Riggs CE, Jr.: Tumor necrosis factor and cytotoxic agents. Effect on squamous carcinoma lines. Arch Otolaryngol Head Neck Surg 116: 436–439, 1990.
35. Giaccone G, Kadoyama C, Maneckjee R, Venzon D, Alexander RB, Gazdar AF: Effects of tumor necrosis factor, alone or in combination with topoisomerase-II-targeted drugs, on human lung cancer cell lines. Int J Cancer 46:326–329, 1990.
36. Iizumi T, Yazaki T, Waku M, Soma G: Immunochemotherapy for murine bladder tumor with a new human recombinant tumor necrosis factor (rTNF-S), VP-16 and hyperthermia. J Urol 142:386–389, 1989.
37. Krosnick JA, Mulé JJ, McIntosh JK, Rosenberg SA: Augmentation of antitumor efficacy by the combination of recombinant tumor necrosis factor and chemotherapeutic agents in vivo. Cancer Res 49:3729–3733, 1989.
38. Bloom ND, Norbergs DA, Sherman B, Sadjadi M, Ramaswamy G, Jacobs R, Ackerman N: Augmentation of the effect of doxorubicin with low-dose tumor necrosis factor in experimental liver metastasis. Mol Biother 2:121–124, 1990.
39. Das AK, Walther PJ, Buckley NJ, Poulton SH: Recombinant human tumor necrosis factor alone and with chemotherapeutic agents. Effect on nude mouse-supported human bladder cancer heterografts. Arch Surg 124:107–110, 1989.
40. Donaldson JT, Keane TE, Poulton SH, Walther PJ: Enhanced in vivo cytotoxicity of recombinant human tumor necrosis factor with etoposide in human renal cell carcinoma. Evaluation in a pre-clinical model. Urol Res 18:245–250, 1990.
41. Burgers JK, Marshall FF, Isaacs JT: Enhanced anti-tumor effects of recombinant human tumor necrosis factor plus VP-16 on metastatic renal cell carcinoma in a xenograft model. J Urol 142:160–164, 1989.
42. Schmid DS, Hornung R, McGrath KM, Paul N, Ruddle NH: Target cell DNA fragmentation is mediated by lymphotoxin and tumor necrosis factor. Lymphokine Res 6: 195–202, 1987.
43. Kyprianou N, English HF, Isaacs JT: Programmed cell death during regression of PC-82 human prostate cancer following androgen ablation. Cancer Res 50:3748–3753, 1990.
44. Rubin BY, Anderson SL, Lunn RM, Hellermann GR, Smith LJ: Fragmentation of cellular DNA is a nonspecific indicator of responsiveness to tumor necrosis factor. J Biol Response Mod 8:553–559, 1989.
45. Kyprianou N, Alexander RB, Isaacs JT: Activation of programmed cell death by recombinant human tumor necrosis factor plus topoisomerase II targeted drugs in L929 cells. J Natl Cancer Inst 83:346–350, 1991.
46. Utsugi T, Mattern MR, Mirabelli CK, Hanna N: Potentiation of topoisomerase inhibitor-induced DNA strand breakage and cytotoxicity by tumor necrosis factor: Enhancement of topoisomerase activity as a mechanism of potentiation. Cancer Res 50:2636–2640, 1990.
47. Taylor C, Hersh E, Plezia P, Alberts D, McCloskey T, Wiggins C, Ahmann F, King D, Rudolph A: A phase I and pharmacokinetic study of recombinant tumor necrosis factor and doxorubicin (abstr.). Proc Am Soc Clin Oncol 8:183–183, 1989.
48. Orr D, Oldham R, Lewis M, Bertoli L, Birch R: Phase I study of the sequenced administration of etoposide and recombinant tumor necrosis factor in patients with advanced malignancy (Abstr.). Proc Am Soc Clin Oncol 8:190–190, 1989.
49. Simons JW, Rowinsky EK, McGuire WP, Fornastiere AA, Nelson WG, Ettinger DS, Grochow LB, Clarke BV, Lubejko BG, Duerr MT, Burgers JK, Marshall FF, Donehower

RG: Phase I study of overlapping continuous infusion VP-16 and recombinant human tumor necrosis factor in advanced cancer (Abstr.). Proc Am Soc Clin Oncol 9:200–200, 1990.
50. Riggs CE, Davis RT, Ratain MJ, Schilsky R, Vogelzang NJ, Geick J, Jarnow L, O'Brien S, Denger P: Pharmacokinetics of adriamycin in combination with human tumor necrosis factor. Results from a phase I trial (Abstr.). Proc Am Assoc Cancer Res 31:179–179, 1990.
51. Kahn JO, Kaplan LD, Volberding PA, Ziegler JL, Crowe S, Saks SR, Abrams DI: Intralesional recombinant tumor necrosis factor-alpha for AIDS-associated Kaposi's sarcoma: A randomized, double-blind trial. J Acquir Immune Defic Syndr 2:217–223, 1989.
52. Bahnson RR, Ballou BT, Ernstoff MS, Cramer DV, Schwentker FN, Reiland JM, Hakala TR: Toxicity of intravesical recombinant human tumor necrosis factor in cynomolgus monkeys. J Biol Response Mod 9:445–447, 1990.
53. Raeth U, Schmid H, Hofman J, Wiedenmann B, Kempeni J, Schlick E, Kaufmann M: Intraperitoneal application of recombinant tumor necrosis factor as an effective palliative treatment of malignant ascites from ovarian and gastroenteropancreatic carcinomas (Abstr.). Proc Am Soc Clin Oncol 8:181–181, 1989.
54. Kasid A, Morecki S, Aebersold P, Cornetta K, Culver K, Freeman S, Director E, Lotze MT, Blaese RM, Anderson WF, Rosenberg SA: Human gene transfer: Characterization of human tumor-infiltrating lymphocytes as vehicles for retroviral-mediated gene transfer in man. Proc Natl Acad Sci USA 87:473–477, 1990.
55. Rosenberg SA, Aebersold P, Cornetta K, Kasid A, Morgan RA, Moen R, Karson EM, Lotze MT, Yang JC, Topalian SL, Merino MJ, Culver K, Miller AD, Blaese RM, Anderson WF: Gene transfer into humans — immunotherapy of patients with advanced melanoma, using tumor-infiltrating lymphocytes modified by retroviral gene transduction. N Engl J Med 323:570–578, 1990.

11. Cell motility as an index of metastatic ability in prostate cancers: Results with an animal model and with human cancer cells

Alan W. Partin, James L. Mohler, and Donald S. Coffey

Many grading systems, both architectural and cytologic, have been developed to assess the metastatic potential of prostate cancers. These quantitative techniques have been applied to the prediction of prognosis based on the study of fixed *dead* cancer cells. Until recently, methods did not exist to enable the study of the dynamic biological properties of *live* cancer cells. Time-lapse videomicroscopy of living cancer cells has revealed that some cancer cells demonstrate dynamic motility processes. Cancer, often called a disease of cell structure, has been recognized histologically by pathologists for over 100 years by its altered morphology. The diversity of cell shape and size among cancer cells, first noted by Virchow in 1863 [1], is still described by pathologists through the static analysis of fixed, *dead* cells and only represents a "freeze-frame" of the more dynamic motility events occurring within the *live* cancer cells.

Preliminary time-lapse studies of cancer cells taken from the Dunning R3327 rat model of prostatic adenocarcinoma demonstrated various distinct types of cell motility, including cell membrane ruffing, pseudopodal extension, undulation, and cell translation. The development and testing of a visual motility grading system of these types of cancer cell motility [2–4] proved an accurate method for predicting prognosis among the Dunning model and established the feasibility for the development of a more quantitative approach. This technique based on a combined temporal-spatial Fourier analysis of cell motility [5] allowed accurate simultaneous measurement of these types of cell motility that correlated well with metastatic potential in this animal model of prostate cancer.

We studied the motility of live cancer cells aspirated directly from 55 human radical prostatectomy specimens [6] with clinically localized prostate cancer. Preliminary investigation of the motility of these live human cancer cells has demonstrated the feasibility and limitations of the use of these methods for grading human urologic cancers.

Lepor, H. and Lawson R.K., (eds.), Therapy for Genitourinary Cancer. ©*1992*
Kluwer Academic Publishers. ISBN 0-7923-1412-3.

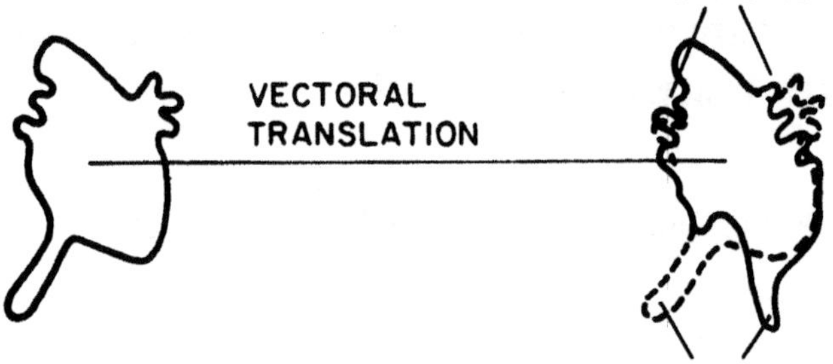

Figure 1. Cell motility grading system. Each parameter of cell motility was graded from 0, none observed, to 5, excessive amounts of motility.

Development and testing of a visual grading system of cell motility

The Dunning R3327 rat prostatic adenocarcinoma tumor model was used to investigate the correlation between cell motility and metastatic potential. The Dunning model, developed from a spontaneous prostatic adenocarcinoma [7], has given rise to several distinct and well-characterized [8] cell-culture variants with differing metastatic potential. Previous biochemical and morphometric attempts at distinguishing among these variants based on metastatic potential have failed [8].

We developed a time-lapse videomicroscopy system [2] with which we studied the motility of live cells from five of the Dunning variants and visually graded six parameters of cell motility, of which three — cell-membrane ruffling, pseudopodal extension, and translation (Figure 1) — contained the information necessary for optimal identification of cells from the various cell lines. Membrane ruffling represents the rapid rhythmic movement of short segments of the cell membrane. Pseudopodal extension represents the extension and retraction of short segments of the cell contour over long distances. Translation represents movement of the cell centroid. This method of grading cell motility proved both accurate and reproducible with intra-assay, intra-observer, and inter-observer reproducilibility of 75%, 80%, and 75%, respectively.

We then tested whether this visual grading system of cell motility could be used to predict the metastatic potential among the various Dunning sublines [3]. Time-lapse films of isolated cells taken from seven (four low metastatic and three highly metastatic) of the Dunning variants were made and visually graded independently under similar conditions by two observers who had no knowledge of the identity of the specimens. The three previously identified parameters — cell membrane ruffling, pseudopodal extension, and translation — were graded subjectively from 0 (no motility) to 5 (excessive motility). The scores from both observers were summed to yield a score from 0 to 10, and the sum of the three were averaged to yield a motility index.

Figure 2 demonstrates the marked differences found between cells taken from the highly metastatic cell lines and those from the low metastatic lines. Table 1 demonstrates the classification accuracy for the individual and combinations of the visual grading parameters for the various Dunning cells on the basis of metastatic potential. Translation allowed the correct classification of 26 of 28 specimens, whereas the combination of translation and pseudopodal extension allowed the correct classification of 27 of the 28 cells studied.

Development of a quantitative method of studying cell motility

Our time-lapse videomicroscopy studies and subjective visual motility grading system demonstrated the ability of the human to recognize, classify, and categorize various types of cell motility that correlate well with metastatic potential in cells from the Dunning model of prostate cancer. Noble [9] pointed out that to merely say that a cell has moved, as the visual motility grading system has done, is to only describe a small portion of the information inherent in the dynamic process of cell motility. An accurate quantitative analysis of cell motility must describe absolute distances, angles, frequencies, speeds, randomness, persistence, and temporal shape change. Cell motility measurements from 0 to 5 were too subjective and lack descriptive labels, such as microns, degrees, and seconds. With this in mind, we

Table 1. Subtypes of motility as predictors of metastatic potential

	Motility Grade			
Motility Parameter	High Met.[a]	Low Met.[b]	Significance (p)[c]	% Correct (n = 28)
Ruffling (RUF)	7.92 ± 0.66	3.75 ± 0.66	<0.01	86%
Pseudopodal extension (PSE)	7.42 ± 0.81	1.81 ± 0.53	<0.001	86%
Translation (TRA)	5.92 ± 0.89	0.38 ± 0.18	<0.0001	93%
RUF + PSE	7.79 ± 0.61	2.78 ± 0.54	<0.0001	89%
RUF + TRA	7.00 ± 0.61	1.06 ± 0.04	<0.0001	89%
TRA + PSE	6.67 ± 0.75	1.09 ± 0.34	<0.0001	96%
Motility index (RUF + PSE + TRA/3)	6.92 ± 0.67	1.96 ± 0.41	<0.0001	93%

[a] Mean ± SEM for cell from each of the high-metastatic Dunning sublines (AT3, MAT-Lu, MAT-LyLu).
[b] Mean ± SEM for cell from each of the low-metastatic Dunning sublines (G, HIF, AT1, AT2).
[c] Probability of separation by Mann-Whitney-Wilcoxon analysis.

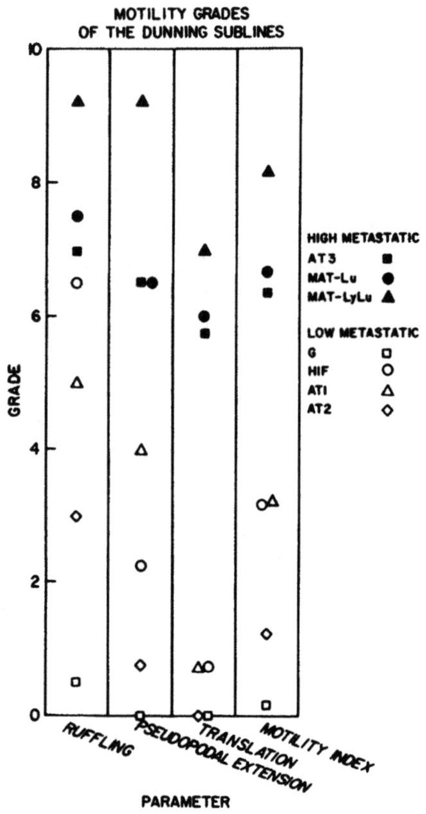

Figure 2. Motility grades of the Dunning sublines. The motility grades for the three motility parameters — ruffling, pseudopodal extension, and translation — as well as the motility index are depicted for seven of the Dunning sublines. Solid figures represent cell lines with ≥90% of sc inoculated animals developing metastases, and open figures represent sublines in which ≤20% of animals develop metastases.

combined the use of timelapse videomicroscopy, image analysis techniques, and a new spatial-temporal two-dimensional Fourier analysis of cell motility to correlate metastatic potential with measurements of cell motility within the Dunning model [5].

The complex shape of a cell contour can be decomposed into spatial harmonics that represent the sinusoidal frequencies that produce that contour. This type of analysis of cell contours utilizes a Fourier transform to provide a mathematical representation of a cell shape by reducing it into its component sine and cosine Fourier coefficients.

Figure 3 demonstrates DynaCELL® (JAW Assoc. Inc., Annapolis, MD), a cell motility, cell morphometry workstation developed based upon this two-dimensional Fourier analysis of cell motility. The prototype of this system was used in the development of this quantitative cell motility technology.

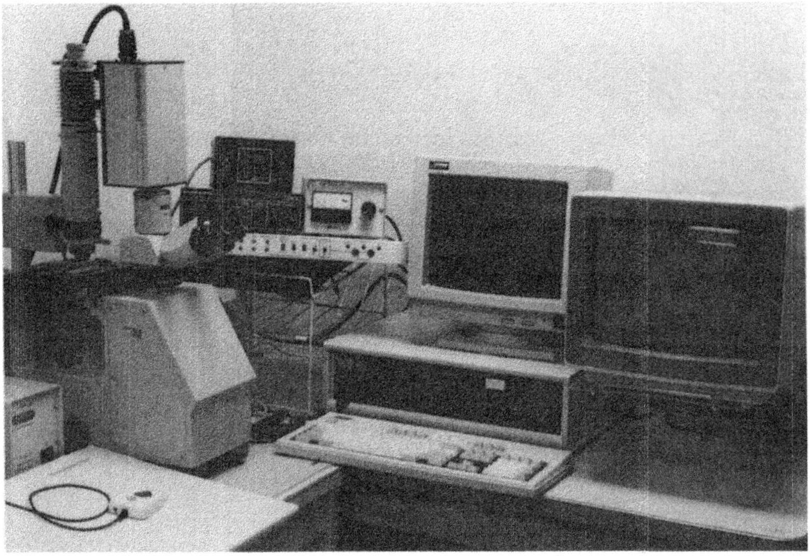

Figure 3. Equipment used for Fourier analysis of cell motility. DynaCELL® (JAW Assoc. Inc., Annapolis, MD). This photograph depicts the equipment used for this new Fourier method of analyzing cell motility. The equipment consists of a computer, frame grabber, VGA monitor, multisync color video monitor, digitizer tablet, Nomarski optics, heated stage, time-date generator, and time controller box.

Figure 4 is a flow diagram depicting the quantitative measurement of cell motility of single cells with a spatial-temporal Fourier analysis of cell motility by this method. Computer-generated models of cell ruffling, pseudopodal extension, undulation, and translation were made. These models were then analyzed with the Fourier technique to determine locations within the Fourier coefficient matrix in which ruffling, undulation, pseudopodal extension, and translation were found. Figure 5 represents a schematic of the two-dimensional diagram of the matrix of Fourier motility coefficients demonstrating the location of the information depicting the various types of cell motility.

We then measured the motility with this method for 26 cells from each of six of the Dunning tumor cell lines with varying metastatic potential. Figure 6 demonstrates the mean and distribution of the various Dunning cell lines, as well as their metastatic potential. The motility coefficients for translation and pseudopodal extension were higher for cells from tumor sublines with higher metastatic potential. Fourier motility coefficients yielded correlation coefficients with a metastatic potential of 0.63 for pseudopodal extension ($p < 0.001$), 0.59 for undulation ($p < 0.001$), 0.50 for translation ($p < 0.001$), and 0.50 for ruffling ($p < 0.001$). This new spatial-temporal Fourier analysis accurately quantifies the different types of cell motility and should aid in the

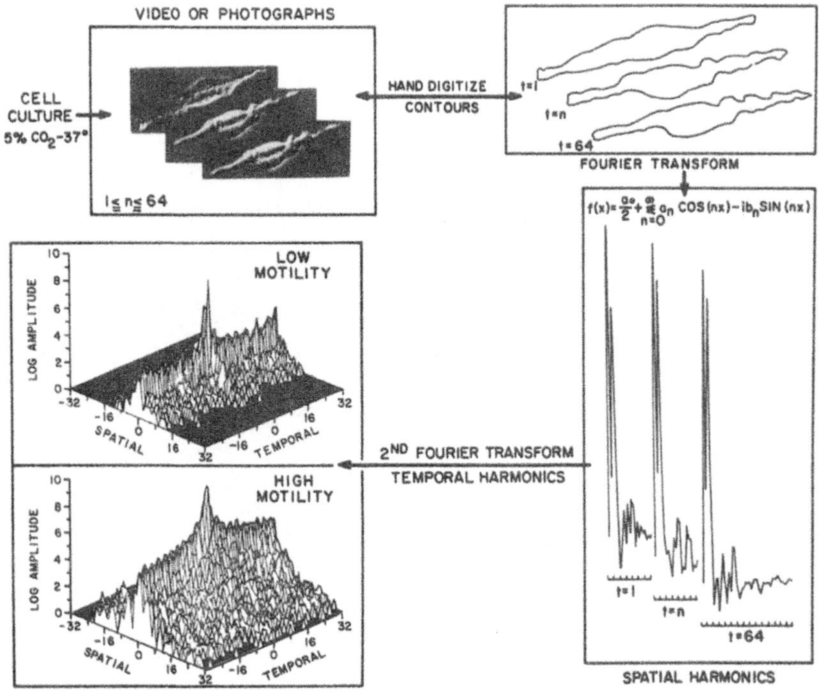

Figure 4. *Left*: Quantitative measurement of the motility of single cells with a spatial-temporal Fourier analysis of time-lapse images. Cells were inoculated at low density on glass. Single cells were viewed at 400x with an inverted Nomarski optics microscope. Images were collected at 60-second intervals for 64 minutes. Cell contours were manually traced with a digitizer tablet in succession. The X-Y coordinates of each successive cell contour were then subject to a spatial complex fast Fourier transform (FFT) to determine the spatial Fourier motility coefficients describing the cell shape. The spatial Fourier coefficients for each of the 64 cell contours were then combined into a matrix and subjected to a second FFT to determine the temporal changes in the spatial Fourier coefficients. The root sum of the square of the coefficient produces the Fourier motility coefficients. This is graphically depicted in a three-dimensional plot. The results of a highly motile cell are compared with that of a low-motile cell.

study of the motility of individual cells in many different areas of cell and tumor biology.

Preliminary studies of visual motility grading with human cells

We investigated the motility of cancer cells taken from 55 radical prostatectomy specimens from patients with clinically localized prostatic carcinoma [6]. Forty-five of the 55 radical prostatectomy specimens yielded adequate attachment to culture plates to allow analysis by time-lapse video-

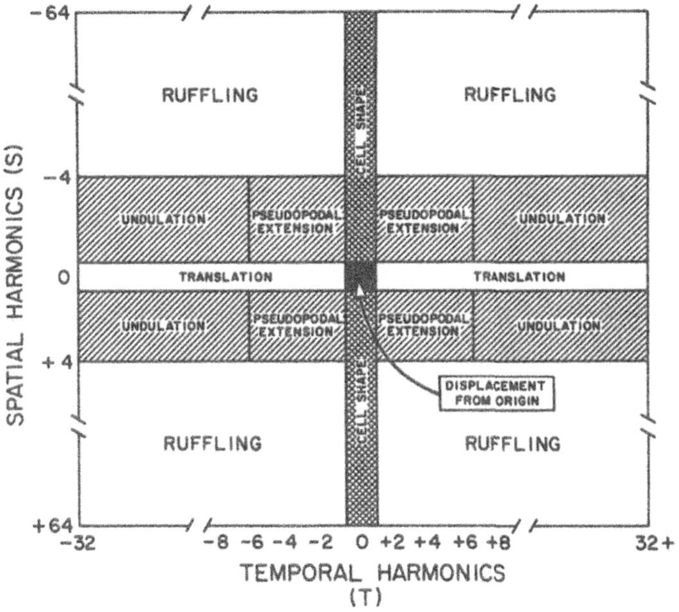

Figure 5. Schematic two-dimensional diagram of the matrix of Fourier motility coefficients. The areas within the matrix contain the Fourier motility coefficients representing ruffling, undulation, pseudopodal extension, and translation.

microscopy for visual grading of the various types of cell motility. This patient group consisted of B1N (6), B1 (28), B2 (10), and C1 (1).

Immediately after removal of the prostatectomy specimen, under sterile conditions, an excisional biopsy of the gross tumor was made and minced into collagenase/trypsin solution for digestion. All cells were plated in identical cell culture media (RPMI 1640) and incubated under standard conditions for 72 hours. One hundred and eighty-six time-lapse video segments were made of the isolated cancer cells (average 3.7 cells per patient studied). The average motility index (sum of the three visual motility parameters) varied markedly within the patients, not only between pathologic grades, but also within a single pathologic grade as well. This separation of patients within and between pathologic grade and stage provides the hope that a motility grading system similar to this may add to the limited ability of stage and grade to predict the prognosis of individual patients with prostatic carcinoma. These early results with human prostatic carcinomas, although too preliminary to ascertain the usefulness as a predictor of progression due to the natural history of this disease, and the fact that only 1 of 45 patients to date has progressed, have in fact demonstrated an increased heterogeneity (coefficient of variation average of 68%) not seen among the cells studied in the Dunning model (coefficient of variations averaging 33%). In summary,

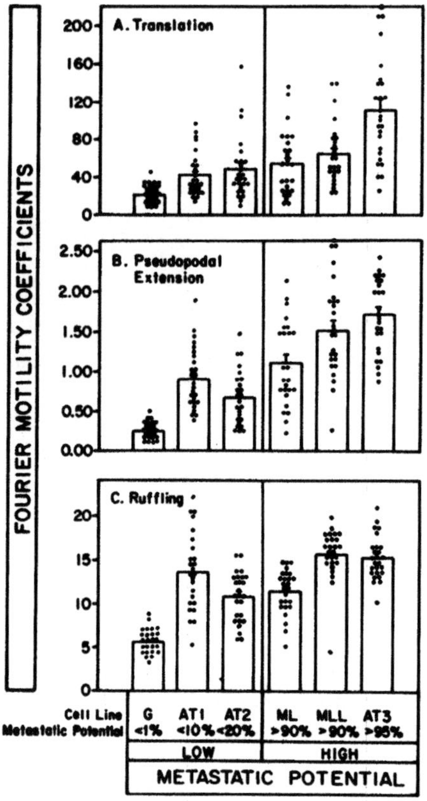

Figure 6. Comparison of the Fourier motility coefficients for translation, pseudopodal extension, and ruffling, for six Dunning cell sublines with varying metastatic potential. Twenty-six cells from each of six Dunning cell lines were analyed with the spatial-temporal Fourier method described in Figures 3 and 4. The metastatic potential of each cell line is expressed as the percent of animals that develop distant metastases following sc injection of 10^5 cells found at the time of death or at autopsy 42 days post-injection. Metastatic potential is arbitrarily defined as low metastatic when <20% of rats develop distant metastases and high when >90% develop distant metastases. Bars represent the mean ± SEM for 26 cells from each cell line. ML and MLL represent MAT-Lu and MAT-LyLu, respectively.

we feel that it is too early to determine the usefulness of cell motility in human prostate cancer, yet we are optimistic that with further research and the use of the quantitative methods previously described, this valuable method of studying the *live* dynamic nature of cancer cells will undoubtedly aid in the study of prostate and other forms of cancer.

Conclusion

Prior to these studies, an accurate method for distinguishing the metastatic potential of the Dunning R3327 rat prostatic adenocarcinoma tumor model did not exist. We developed and tested a visual grading method of cell motility that for the first time was able to distinguish between these cell lines based on their metastatic potential. When tested in a blinded and prospective fashion, this method proved far more accurate than those tested previously.

We feel that examination of *live* cancer cells from human prostatic cancers will undoubtedly provide more information about the biological behavior of these malignancies than the present routine pathologic analysis of *dead* cells. This method, which proved accurate for the Dunning animal model, was tested on human prostate cancer cells in a large group of 45 patients with clinically localized prostate cancer. These preliminary results demonstrated the feasibility and limitations of this methodology for the investigation of human cancers. These methods and others that involve the study of the dynamic properties of *live* cancer cells with prove valuable in the development of more accurate methods for the prediction of metastatic potential in prostate cancer.

Acknowledgments

We thank Dr. Patrick C. Walsh for his support during this project. We thank James Gurganus, Robert Pitcock, Don Vindivich, Susan Dalrymple, and Alexander Walsh for the expert collection and analysis of cell data. We thank Drs. Stephen Piantadosi, John T. Isaacs, William B. Isaacs, Joseph Schoeniger, William Guier, and Mr. Robert Jernigan and Mr. Charles Wheatley for their expert advice. This work was supported by Grant CA 15416 from the National Cancer Institute. A.W.P. was supported through the M.D. Ph.D. Medical Scientist Training Program Grant 5T32 GM07309.

References

1. Virchow R: Ueber bewegliche thierische zellen. Arch Patholo Anat Physiol Klini Medi 28:237–240, 1863.
2. Mohler JL, Partin AW, Isaacs WI, Coffey DS: Time-lapse videomicroscopic identification of Dunning R3327 adenocarcinoma and normal rat prostate cells. J Urol 137:544–547, 1987.
3. Mohler JL, Partin AW, Coffey DS: Prediction of metastatic potential by a new grading system of cell motility: Validation in the Dunning R3327 prostatic adenocarcinoma model. J Urol 138:168–170, 1987.
4. Mohler JL, Partin AW, Isaacs JT, Coffey DS: Metastatic potential prediction by a visual grading system of cell motility: Prospective validation in the Dunning R3327 prostatic adenocarcinoma model. Cancer Res 48:4312–4317, 1988.
5. Partin AW, Schoeniger JS, Mohler JL, Coffey DS: Fourier analysis of cell motility: Correlation of motility with metastatic potetial. Proc Natl Acad Sci USA 86:1254–1258, 1989.
6. Mohler JL, Partin AW, Coffey DS: Cancer cell motility: A visual grading system for assessment of prognosis in prostatic cancer. In: Karr, JP, Coffey DS, Gardner W Jr. (eds). *Prognostic Cytometry and Cytopathology of prostate Cancer*. Elsevier, New York, pp. 337–348.

7. Dunning WF: Prostate cancer in the rat. Natl Cancer Inst Mono 12:351–369, 1963.
8. Isaacs JT, Isaacs WB, Feitz WFJ, Scheres J: Establishment and characterization of seven Dunning rat prostatic cancer cell lines and their use in developing methods for predicting metastatic abilities of prostatic cancers. The Prostate 9:261–281, 1986.
9. Nobel PB: *Computer-Assisted Analysis of Cell Locomotion and Chemotaxis*. CRC Press, Boca Raton, FL, 1986.

12. Suramin as an archetypical compound in the development of growth factor antagonists for inhibition of genitourinary tumors

Howard I. Scher and Warren D.W. Heston

Historical background

Suramin is one of the first synthetic chemotherapeutic agents to be discovered that was clinically effective against a human parasite. The road to its discovery began in 1899 when Paul Ehrlich was appointed director of the Institute for Experimental Therapy in Frankfurt, a time in which the German chemical industry was synthesizing many compounds, including a large number of synthetic dyes. One such dye, trypan red, was shown to cure trypanosomiasis in mice in 1904, the first time a parasitic infection was cured with a chemotherapeutic agent. Trypanosomes that excluded the dye were resistant [1].

Although clinical trials failed to show efficacy in human trypanosomal disease, trypan red did serve as the precursor for the structurally related compound, suramin, which entered trial in 1920 [2]. Suramin is effective in early- but not late-stage (central nervous system) trypanosomisis and the filarial infection onchocerciasis. Poor central nervous system penetration probably explains the absence of an effect in the later stages of the disease, which is very selective for this structure [2]. Even minor deviations result in a loss of activity [3]. In 1930, the compound was shown to be active in treating the autoimmune disorder pemphigus [4], and it was during these trials that the toxic effects on the adrenal cortex were first recognized [4,5]. In addition to being an adrenal toxin, suramin inhibits steroid hormone production [6].

Interest in the compound was renewed in 1979 when the inhibitory effects on nucleic acid polymerases and the reverse transcriptase of RNA tumor viruses were recognized [7]. This, coupled with observation that suramin could reduce viremia in patients with AIDS, led to clinical trials in this disease. Although the trials were negative [8], regression of a Kaposi's sarcoma, a tumor known to be associated with autocrine production of fibroblast growth factor (FGF), was observed [9]. The putative effects of suramin on growth factor activity have generated the greatest interest in the compound.

Lepor, H. and Lawson R.K., (eds.), Therapy for Genitourinary Cancer. *ISBN 0-7923-1412-3.*

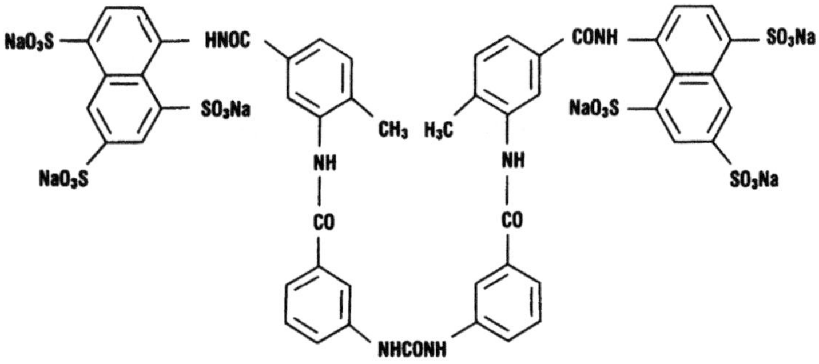

Figure 1. The structure of sodium suramin.

Mechanisms of action

Suramin, a polysulfonated napthylurea (M.W. 1429 daltons), is the hexa-sodium salt of 8,8′-(carbonylbis(imino-3,1-phenylenecarbonylimino(4-methyl-3,1phenylene)carbonylimino)bis-1,3,5-napthylenetrisulfonic acid (Figure 1). Based on its polyanionic structure, a high degree of nonspecific protein binding, primarily to basic compounds, is anticipated. In plasma, over 99% is protein bound [10]. It does exhibit a degree of specificity, as does the related compound, heparin. It is also related structurally to trypan blue, a compound that is actively excluded by living cells and is used in tests of cell viability. At present it is unclear whether the principal actions of suramin are extracellular, inhibiting the action of polypeptide growth factors to their receptors [3], or intracellular (*vide infra*).

One of the mechanisms of tumorigenic transformation is the inappropriate secretion of growth factors. In some instances, these growth factors bind to and activate their own growth factor receptors, thereby inducing cellular division. This is termed *autocrine growth factor production*. One of the first oncogenes to be identified and cloned was the *v-sis* oncogene, later shown to be similar to the normal cellular growth factor platelet-derived growth factor, PDGF. Because of suramin's polyanionic character, it was examined as a potential inhibitor of the action of PDGF, a protein with a preponderance of basic amino acids and an isoelectric point of nearly 10. Suramin was subsequently shown to bind directly to PDGF, to displace receptor-bound PDGF, and to prevent PDGF-induced mitogenesis of PDGF-responsive cells [11,12]. Cells that are chronically stimulated by autocrine growth factor production often exhibit a lower number of cell-surface receptors for that growth factor than their normal counterparts. This is believed to be the result of internalization of the growth-factor receptor, with subsequent down-regulation of the surface receptor. In simian sarcoma virus-transformed cells (*v-sis*), the number of PDGF receptors are decreased relative to their nontransformed counterparts. Treatment with suramin results in an increase in the number of cell-surface receptors [13]. The transformed appearance of the cells also reverts to normal [14].

Huang and Huang reported that *sis*-transformed cell PDGF receptors are activated intracellularly and thus never reach the surface before being activated and down-regulated, providing one reason for the decreased number of receptors in these transformed cells. They determined that suramin would block this intracellular autocrine loop and postulated that suramin could also act intracellularly [15].

The ability of suramin to inhibit growth factor binding in vitro correlates well with its ability to inhibit cell growth as measured by the inhibition of DNA synthesis, as well as by assays of cell number and colony forming ability. This has been shown for a number of cell lines in vitro. The reported results must be interpreted carefully however, as ID50s can vary with 1) the concentration of suramin, 2) the serum concentration in the medium, 3) the number and type of cells plated, and 4) the duration of exposure. The latter may be critical to optimal clinical use of the compound. For example, a suramin concentration that had minimal effect on EGF-induced mitogenesis of AKR-2B cells, blocked EGF mitogenesis on LNCaP cells by over 90% [17]. Coffey and coworkers examined the effect of suramin on the binding of basic fibroblast growth factor (b-FGF), transforming growth factor-beta (TGF-β), and epidermal growth factor (EGF) to specific receptors in AKR-2B fibroblasts [16]. An inhibition of both growth factor binding and growth factor-induced mitogenic activity on transformed and nontransformed cells was reported. However, a significant variation in the ID50 for each growth factor was observed. For example, b-FGF was 33 and 40 times more sensitive to inhibition than EGF for the binding and mitogenic activities respectively. A compilation of these effects is denoted in Table 1. Increasing

Table 1. Effect of suramin on growth factor binding and mitogenic activity: ID_{50} concentration of suramin

Mitogen	Growth-Factor Binding	^{3}H-TTP Thymidine
b-FGF (16)	0.015 mM	.01 mM
TGF-β	0.03 mM	.01 mM
PDGF (12)	0.06 mM	.08 mM
EGF	0.50 mM	.40 mM
Insulin (14)	>0.13 mM	>.13 mM
Ca^{2+}	>0.13 mM	>.13 mM

Data interpolated from figures in refs. 16 (bFGF, TGF-β), 12 (EGF, PDGF, insulin), and 14 (calcium) as the concentration in millimoles required to reduce by 50% the binding of the growth factor to its receptor or to inhibit ^{3}H-thymidine incorporation into DNA (ID_{50} = inhibitory dose 50).

concentrations of albumin may abrogate suramin action [18]. In general, inhibitory effects in the range of 200–300 μg/ml (133–200 μM), the therapeutic window for clinical use [19], are considered desirable for further investigation. In most cell lines studied, inhibition of b-FGF-, TGF-β-, and PDGF-related functions occur in this concentration range.

TGF-β represents a family of multifaceted homologous proteins in which the nine cysteine residues are conserved. It also includes other more distantly related peptides that share significant sequence homology [20]. In general, the TFG-β family — TGF-β_1,β_2,β_3 — bind to the same three receptors that are differentially distributed in different tissues. Stimulation by TGF-β tends to increase extracellular matrix components; increases cell adhesion molecules, such as the fibronectin receptor; decreases the synthesis of proteinases, such as cathepsin and collagenase; and increases the synthesis of tissue proteinase inhibitors. It is believed to play a major role in wound and tissue repair, bone formation and remodeling, and embryogenesis. Many of its functions are associated with growth inhibition, and TGF-β is the most potent known growth inhibitor for a wide variety of cell types of mesenchymal, myeloid, epithelial, lymphoid, and endothelial origin. Some tumors are thought to have become growth deregulated because they have lost their ability to respond to TGF-β. In instances where TGF-β is associated with mitogenic activity, it may be due to the stimulation of PDGF production by TGF-β [21]. For some systems, blocking TGF-β action in vivo may result in the release of a negative growth control and result in increased, as opposed to decreased, tumor growth. TGF-β has been isolated from conditioned media of prostate cancer cell lines [22], and functional receptors have been described [23]. Both positive and negative effects have been observed [23]. Because of the many cellular interactions involved in the growth of solid tumors and the many functions of TGF-β, it may be that blocking of TGF-β paracrine, rather than autocrine, interactions are responsible for its activity.

Basic fibroblast growth factor (bFGF) has also been shown to be inhibited by suramin in concentrations that are achievable clinically. Like TGF-β, FGF has a wide range of actions on many cell types [24,25]. These include an increase in cell growth, induction of plasminogen activator, an increase in type IV collagenase activity, and increased cell migration. In vivo, bFGF causes neovascularization, induces fibroplasia of the dermis, and induces differentiation of the mesenchyme in embryonic tissue [24]. The induction of differentiation of embryonic mesenchyme can be inhibited by heparin. FGF lacks a classical signal sequence, and it is unclear how it is secreted from the cell. It may only be released during cell death. Cells transformed by FGF demonstrate no extracellular FGF, and it is hypothesized that the FGF acts via an intracellular autocrine mechanism [25]. In a series of experiments, it was shown that transfection of bFGF fused to an immunoglobulin signal-peptide sequence resulted in increased proliferation, increased cell density, and anchorage-independent growth. Cell-surface receptors were decreased, and growth was not inhibited by antibodies to the FGF receptor. Treatment with suramin up-regulates the receptors and reverts the transformed phenotype [26]. Some members of the FGF-like family of proteins, such as int-2, Hst/K-fgf, and FGF-5, do have regions associated with secretion. Transfectants of these other FGFs secrete the protein and exhibit transformation at much lower levels of production of the FGF-like protein [24]. Moscatelli and colleagues found that the number of fgf receptors were decreased by transfection with the *hst/K-fgf* oncogene for transformation. Treatment with suramin reversed the transformation and restored the receptor number [27]. Two receptors for FGF have been described using photoaffinity labelling experiments. Acidic FGF preferentially binds to one and b-FGF to the other. Each is able to displace the other.

Members of the FGF family have a strong affinity for heparin, which was exploited for isolation and purification. Extracellular FGF binds to the extracellular matrix, especially heparan sulfate proteoglycans [24]. This may act as a storage form of FGF, and studies suggest that binding to the matrix may prolong the action of FGF, a so-called stormone. For example, stimulation of plasminogen activator was more prolonged and intense in cells stimulated by FGF and washed with HBSS than in cells in which the FGF was not only washed but was stripped from the extracellular matrix [20]. The action of heparan sulfact proteoglycans in the stroma of the bone marrow is similar. These compounds help to localize heparin-binding colony-stimulating factors, such as granulocyte macrophage colony stimulating factor (GM-CSF), to the stromal matrix where the interaction with stem cells occurs [28].

Platelet-derived growth factor (PDGF) is also inhibited by suramin, but usually requires higher concentrations than those needed to inhibit TGF-β and FGF [11]. PDGF is associated with the growth of mesenchymal tissues and probably is not involved in autocrine growth of urologic adenocarcinomas. It may be involved in paracrine, rather than autocrine, actions in these tumors. As noted previously, TGF-β will induce PDGF, and one aspect of suramin's action is that it will block both of these actions.

Growth factors and the prostate

Prostate cancer cell growth is mediated by a number of factors in addition to androgen. While the mechanisms involved in the development of androgen escape are not completely understood, it has been postulated that autocrine production of growth factors that previously required the presence of steroid for their production may contribute. In the prostate, a number of growth factors have been identified, including basic and acidic FGF, EGF, and transforming growth factors alpha and beta [29–31]. While the actions and interactions of these factors are complex, and the relative contribution of each factor is unknown, fibroblast growth factors seem to be present in

Table 2. Content of growth-factor activity and percentage of heparin-binding growth factor in extracts of normal, BPH, and cancerous human prostates (CAP), both untreated and following DES treatment for cancer [26, 27]

	Hierowski [26]		Nishi [27]	
Prostatic Cytosol[a]	Units/mg prot.	%HiA[b]	Units/mg prot.	%HiA
Normal	44 ± 14	8%	158 ± 52	84%
BPH	195 ± 34[c]	90%[c]	660 ± 389[c]	95%
CAP	208 ± 39[c]	95%[c]	317 ± 76[c]	88%
CAP & DES	—		164 ± 94[d]	91%

[a] Normals were obtained following autopsy of young men, (n = 4) (Hierowski), or cystoprostatectomy for bladder cancer or autopsy (n = 2 & 2) of older men (Nishi). Nishi obtained BPH (n = 6) and CAP (n = 3) specimens following open prostatectomy procedures, and the DES patients (n = 9) received diethylstilbestrol phosphate (0.3–0.5 g/day) for 2–4 weeks before prostatectomy. Values represent mean ± SD.
[b] HiA represents the percentage of growth-factor activity that exhibited high affinity for heparin as defined by binding to heparin in the presence of 0.5 M NaCl.
[c] $p < .05$ vs. normal control.
[d] $p < .05$ vs. CAP control.

the highest relative proportion. FGF-like growth factor activity from rat and human prostates has been assessed in biological assays using 3T3 fibroblasts, MC3T3-E1 osteoblasts, endothelial cells, and prostate epithelial cells as targets. All of these data suggest a role for FGF in the angiogenesis, stromal growth, osteoblastic growth, and malignant prostatic epithelial cell growth in vivo (Table 2) [32–38].

Nishi et al. and Hierowski and coworkers have used heparin binding to determine the relationship between the percentage of heparin-binding growth-factor activity and the presence of benign prostatic hypertrophy or prostatic cancer relative to the normal prostate. The effect of diethylstilbesterol (DES) pretreatment on the amount of growth factor activity was also examined [37,38]. An increased amount of growth factor activity was observed in BPH relative to malignant specimens. The absolute levels of activity are different and may be the result of differences in the bioassay used. Differences were also observed with age. In young men, 92% of the activity isolated was not heparin binding [37]. The opposite was observed in an older population [38], suggesting that increased levels of FGF may correlate with aging. Treatment with DES resulted in a decrease in both the units of activity per milligram of protein and the total activity in the prostate. The total units per gram of prostate decreased from 11,100 ± 2500 to 6300 ± 3800 for the DES-treated group, close to the 4300 ± 1900 for the normal prostates studied. The amount of activity decreased to normal levels in 8 of 10 (80%) cases [38]. It was not stated whether the two cases that did not return to normal were in fact unresponsive to DES therapy. The decreased levels with hormone therapy are consistent with the possibility that FGF is one of the autocrine/paracrine growth regulators of the human prostate.

The LNCaP human prostatic carcinoma cell line was originally isolated by Horoszewicz [39]. It produces prostatic acid phosphatase and prostatic-specific antigen, and was used to produce the new prostatic marker CYT 356, that has shown immunoreactivity with virtually all of the prostatic tumors examined [40]. It has receptors for androgens and sublines have been isolated that are growth stimulated by dihydrotestosterone. Using a LNCaP cell line obtained from Steve Harris of the Alton Jones Cell Science Center in Lake Placid, New York, we examined the effect of suramin in inhibiting the growth of the LNCaP line in the presence and absence of dihydrotestosterone. The interaction of tumor necrosis factor (TNF), noted to cause cell death of carcinoma cells, and of dexamethasone were also evaluated. TNF was examined because of its growth-suppressing effects on the LNCaP line, while dexamethasone was evaluated because patients treated with suramin require steroid replacement because of the adrenocortical toxicities of the compound.

Binding studies with radiolabeled TNF showed that suramin (100 μM) had no effect on the binding of TNF to the high-affinity receptor on LNCaP cells. To reduce the endogenous steroid content, the experiments were performed in charcoal-stripped serum. In this study, 3×10^4 LNCaP cells in 5% charcoal-stripped serum in DME:HAMSF-12 1:1 were supplemented with insulin, transferrin, and selenium (ITS). Twenty-four hours later, suramin (100 μM), TNF (1 nM), dihydrotestosterone (20 nM), and/or dexamethasone were added. The results are shown in Table 3.

Treatment with suramin was very effective in blocking the growth induced by DHT, consistent with its growth-factor antagonistic action. During this 7-day exposure, cell growth was antagonized, but the over-

Table 3. The effect of suramin (100 μM) and TNF (1 μM) in the presence or absence of 20 μM of dihydrotestosterone (DHT) or dexamethasone (DEX) on the growth of LNCaP cells

	Cell # ($\times 10^4$)		
Treatment	—	+DHT	+DEX
Control	27.6 ± 1.4[a]	46.5 ± 2.5	29.6 ± 2.6
Suramin	11.7 ± 0.9	15.5 ± 3.2	14.0 ± 1.4
TNF	16.0 ± 0.4	31.5 ± 1.7	18.2 ± 2.1
SUR + TNF	4.6 ± 0.4	5.8 ± 2.0	4.9 ± 1.3

[a] Values represent the mean ± SD. All values of the individual treatments differed significantly from the controls, as well as the combined treatment.

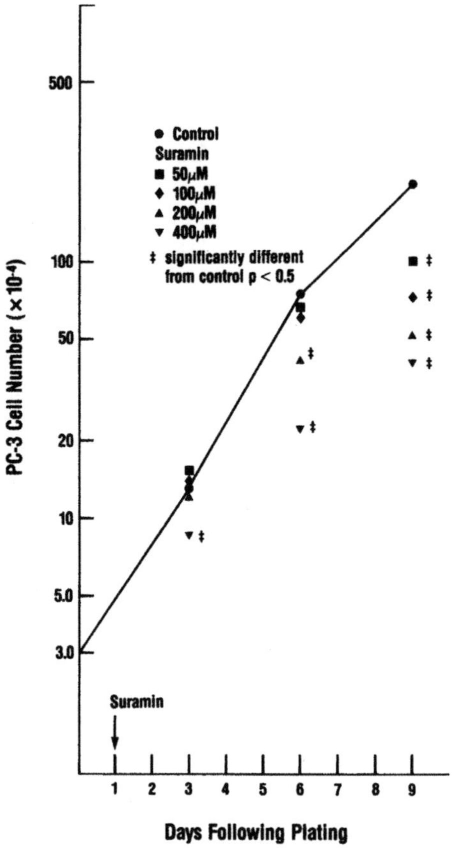

Figure 2. Thirty thousand PC-3 cells were plated and the following day different concentrations of suramin were added to the cells. The exposure to the suramin was for the time periods shown, after which the cells were removed from the plate and counted.

all cell number was not reduced, consistent with a cytostatic effect. TNF was less effective in inhibiting the growth of DHT-stimulated cells relative to cells grown in the charcoal-stripped serum. Combining TNF and suramin produced additive effects that were not reversed by the addition of dihydrotestosterone or dexamethasone. Other have also observed TNF to be growth suppressive to LNCaP lines [41]. The results, however, must be interpreted cautiously because of deficiencies in the LNCaP model. LNCaP lacks receptors for TGFβ, an inhibitor of cell growth, so the effect of suramin on TGFβ in this system cannot be determined [29,42]. The LNCaP cells also have a mutated androgen receptor that permits the binding of other steroids, in particular, progestins. Some prostatic epithelial cells have been shown to be inhibited by glucocorticoids. Unrecognized differences in the androgen receptor may result in differential glucocorticoid responses in some LNCaP variants.

Table 4. Effect of prolonged exposure to suramin on PC-3 cells

Treatment	Cell No. ($\times 10^4$)
Plated day 0	1.0
Control day 6	16.6 ± 1.0
Suramin day 6	9.4 ± 1.0
Rinsed day 12	56.2 ± 2.3
Suramin day 12	1.2 ± 0.1

Ten thousand PC-3 cells were plated. The following day, 100 μM suramin was added, and 5 days later (6 days following plating), the cells were counted or the cells were rinsed, fresh media was added, and the incubation continued with or without the presence of 100 μM suramin.

We also examined the effect of suramin on the growth of the PC-3 human prostatic cancer cell line. The concentration times time (c × t) dose response of these cells to the growth-suppressive effects of suramin are noted in Figure 2. As expected with an increase in either concentration or time of exposure, an increased growth-suppressive effect is observed. The importance of the time of exposure to suramin is also shown in Table 4. If cells are rinsed free of suramin after 5 days of exposure, cytostatic effects are reversed and cell growth resumes. In contrast, if the exposure is continued, cytotoxicity is observed. As illustrated, cell number decreased an additional 82% (9.4 to 1.2×10^4) with continued exposure. Histologic examination of the cells at day 12 was consistent was a cytotoxic effect. The effects of suramin on PC-3 cells have also been shown to be dependent on the concentration of serum in the medium. In one report, the IC50 increased tenfold (from 30 to 300 μM) as the concentration of serum was increased from 2 to 10% [43]. A similar cytostatic effect of increasing serum concentrations was shown using DU-145 cells exposed for 4 hours. Cell growth was inhibited after 3 days. Histologic examination showed irreversible mitochondrial damage, which may be a measure of the toxic effects of the drug [44]. These data also support the complexity of growth-factor interactions in these systems.

Mitchen et al. studied primary human prostate epithelial cultures. Mitogenic effects were reversible up to 6 days, beyond which cytotoxicity was observed. Growth inhibition was seen at suramin concentrations $>10^{-4}$ M. Concentrations in the range of 5×10^{-7} to 10^{-5} M stimulated growth in 9 out of 14 cultures [45]. Mixed responses have also been noted in the Dunning tumor model. Morton et al. studied the effects of suramin on the R3327-AT-2 variant of the Dunning prostatic carcinoma cell line. Growth inhibition was observed [46]. In contrast, we have observed growth stimulation of the Dunning R3327-AT-3 and MAT-LYLU variants (Table 5). These data suggest that removal of inhibitory influences may have adverse effects on cell growth and may possibly accelerate the disease. This may have therapeutic implications.

Table 5. The effect of different doses of suramin on the growth of the R3327MAT-LYLU prostate-derived tumor cell line

Treatment	Cell No. ($\times 10^5$)
Control	41.8 ± 0.8
50 μM suramin	41.2 ± 2.3
100 μM suramin	45.3 ± 1.1
200 μM suramin	58.9 ± 2.7
400 μM suramin	70.3 ± 1.9

Three hundred thousand MAT-LYLU cells were plated. The next day suramin at the different concentrations was added, and 5 days after plating the number of cells were determined by Coulter counting. Two hundred and 400 μM levels of suramin significantly increased the number of cells recovered.

Other non-growth factor activities

The observation that increased durations of exposure to suramin are cytotoxic raises the question of whether prolonged growth factor deprivation is responsible. Often the presence of growth factor antagonists will prevent cells from growing yet will not be cytotoxic. Is the reason that long exposures are required because of the delayed uptake of the highly charged molecule, or are other actions of suramin responsible? Suramin has been shown to inhibit a number of enzymes, including nucleic acid polymerases [47]. It disrupts the activity of a number of membrane-associated ion pumps, such as NaK, Ca, and H^+-ATPases [48,49]. Suramin was also observed to block signal-transducing mechanisms, such as specific G binding proteins and protein kinase C [50,51]. The effects on signal-transduction signaling are not due to an effect on receptor binding. Both opioid and fetal calf serum stimulated high-affinity GTPase activity in a pertussis toxin-sensitive manner that is due to different G proteins. Suramin completely inhibited the opioid-stimulated GTPase activity without affecting the serum-stimulated activity in signal transduction, suggesting a suramin selective effect on these G proteins [50]. Hensey and coworkers examined the inhibitory activity of suramin towards purified protein kinase C. Suramin was a competitive inhibitor with a K_i of 10 μM relative to ATP. They postulated that suramin could be causing inhibition of the growth and inducing differentiation of the NB-2 cells via an effect on PKC. This mechanism, however, would require an intracellular localization of the compound. In the HT29 colon cell line, suramin inhibits cell growth and induces differentiation, an effect felt to be due to its inhibition of an autocrine growth factor [52–54]. In both cases, however, the effect is not immediate but takes several days to occur. It is possible that some uptake has occurred by this time and that some of suramin's activity is due in part to the inhibition of these intracellular processes.

While the focus of suramin's action has been at the cell surface, another aspect of suramin's action takes place in the lysosomal environment. Suramin inhibits lysosomal function, resulting at least in part from its binding and inhibition of various enzymes, such as hyaluronidase, iduronate sulfatase, β-glucuronidase, and sphingoid hydrolases [55,56]. Iduronate synthetase is the most sensitive. Suramin accumulates in the lysosomes of the reticuloendothelial system and in the proximal tubules of the kidney [3]. The inhibition of lysosomal enzyme synthesis results in a systemic accumulation of glycosoaminoglycans (GAGs) and sphingolipids, mimicking the pathology associated with mucopolysaccharidosis [57]. GAGs, primarily heparan and dermatan sulfate, accumulate in the serum, urine, kidney, liver, lung, and spleen [3,55,57]. It also inhibits H^+-ATPase, thus altering the pH gradient of the endosomes, lysosomes, and the processes associated with endocytosis [49,50].

The alterations in GAGs may prove to be of major importance for the activity of suramin. In one report, a temporal relationship between the development of anticoagulation (serum circulating heparans and dermatans) and tumor shrinkage was suggested [19]. The same group reported a fivefold increase in urinary glycosaminoglycans following suramin and have observed that these glycosoaminoglycans were toxic to human adrenal (SW-13) and prostatic (LNCaP) cells, whereas heparan isolated from normal kidney was not toxic [58].

Clinical trials

Pharmacology

As expected for a highly charged molecule, orally administered suramin is poorly absorbed from the intestine. Most clinical investigations have used intravenous dosing schedules. Following intravenous injection, suramin binds to a variety of plasma proteins, such as albumin, globulins, and fibrinogen, with little evidence of diffusion into red blood cells [3]. Over 99.7% is protein bound and no reproducible assay for "free" vs. "bound" suramin is generally available [11]. There is no evidence for a metabolic transformation of suramin [2]; renal excretion accounts for most of its elimination [3]. Suramin appears to be filtered through the renal glomeruli and then reabsorbed by the cells of the proximal tubule. Because the therapeutic window is narrow, 200–300 µg/ml [19], *vide infra*, plasma concentration monitoring is essential [59]. Several assay methods have been published, including one based on an extraction procedure [60] and a second based on direct injection on a high-pressure liquid chromatography column followed by isocratic elution [61]. The latter has the advantage of rapid turnaround times.

Initial clinical trials used a weekly intravenous dose schedule. This proved to be too toxic, and subsequently continuous infusion schedules were studied. At the NCI, patients received a 200-mg test dose followed by a continuous infusion of 350 mg/m^2/day. Treatments were continued until plasma concentrations reached 280–300 µg/ml [19]. Due to the toxic effects on the adrenal glands [5,8], all patients received hydrocortisone replacement therapy from the start of treatment. A nomogram was derived for weekly dose adjustments based on measured plasma concentrations. The median time to achieve therapeutic levels varied from 1 to 4 weeks, and the planned interval between treatment cycles, 2–3 months, was based on the published literature half-life of 55 days [11].

Our initial investigations in patients with bidimensionally measurable prostatic cancer with the same dose schedule showed a similar variation in the time to achieve therapeutic concentrations. Of concern, however, was the observation of a much shorter half-life than previously reported, ranging from 15–39 days. Subsequently, a data-sparse adaptive feedback control algorithm to optimize individual patient treatments was developed. Using published literature values and derived pharmacokinetic parameters in our patient population, a maximum *a posteriori* Bayesian (MAP-B) PK parameter value estimator was implemented [62]. Using this technique, samples drawn on day 1 and 2 are used to predict concentrations on day 3, etc. Dosing recommendations for both continuous IV (one sample on days 1, 2, 3, and 5, then q3D until day 14) and for an intermittent bolus regimen were derived [63]. An example of the measured and predicted plasma concentrations for a patient treated with continuous infusion is illustrated in Figure 3. As shown, the patient was retreated when trough levels reached 100 µg/ml. Other groups have used a fixed dose until therapeutic levels are achieved [64,65].

The combined literature and derived data showed that the plasma disposition of the total drug can be characterized by a two-compartment model. However, as shown in Table 6, considerable variation is evident. The model shows that for the first 2 weeks of therapy, net clearance from the plasma is dominated by the distributional clearance, CL_D [63,66]. As a pseudo-equilibrium between peripheral tissues and plasma is approached, the net clearance from the plasma decreases and approaches the steady-state minimum or total plasma clearance CL_T. Thus, if the therapeutic goal is to rapidly achieve and then to maintain a target plasma suramin concentration,

Table 6. Pharmacokinetic parameters based on literature values and derived MAP-Bayesian estimator [10, 63]

Volume of the central compartment	$V_c = 3.7$ l/m^2
Total steady-state volume	$V_{ss} = 10–25$ l/m^2
Distributional clearance	$CL_D = 0.5–2.5$ l/day/m^2
Distributional half-life	$t_{1/2}a = 0.5–3$ days
Total plasma clearance	$CL_T = 0.3–0.7$ l/day/m^2
Terminal elimination half-life	$t_{1/2}b = 15–55$ days

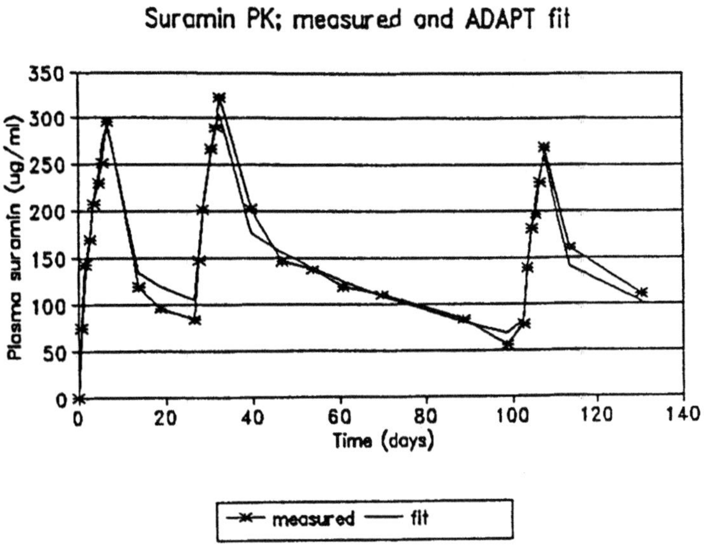

Figure 3. Predicted (*) and measured (+) plasma suramin concentrations using the MAP-Bayesian estimator [63] in a patient with measurable prostatic cancer treated with a continuous-infusion dose schedule.

an "ideal" regimen would require an initial loading dose to load the central compartment, followed by a rapid dose rate that tapers over time to a final steady state. The method of acheiving the target concentration may not be as critical as the use of intermittent doses to maintain concentrations for longer durations.

Toxicity profile

Administration of suramin is different than traditional chemotherapy, as several unique toxicities are observed. Most are mediated by the effects of suramin on glycosaminoglycan synthesis or growth factor inhibition. The most worrisome toxicity is a progressive polyradiculopathy, which can progress to a Guillain-Barre syndrome. The risk is related to peak levels of the compound, increasing rapidly as levels exceed 300 μg/ml, and exceeds 40% at levels above 350 μg/ml [67]. A clear effect of the duration of exposure has not been established. Electromyography and nerve-conduction studies showed evidence of conduction block, suggestive of a demyelinating polyneuropathy. The inhibitory effect of suramin on FGF, a growth factor for Schwann cells, has been postulated.

Suramin is taken up and accumulates in the lysosomes, especially Kupffer cells of the liver and the cortex of the kidney [3]. These two tissues also exhibit toxicity following suramin therapy. Liver-function test abnormalities are observed, especially in individuals with an underlying hepatic insult, such as chronic alcohol abuse, or extensive hepatic involvement by tumor [3]. Proteinuria and decreases in renal clearance have been observed. This may be related to the selective accumulation of suramin in the kidney [68].

A coagulopathy, due to circulating glycosaminoglycans such as heparan and chondroitan sulfate, has been reported. These compounds function as circulating anticogulants. Although serious bleeding has been observed, discontinuation of the drug leads to normalization of the coagulation parameters in several days. Most clinical protocols include provisions to discontinue suramin infusions if the prothrombin time exceeds 17 seconds [69,70].

A vortex keratopathy has been observed in up to 25% of cases [3]. Symptoms include blurring of vision, tearing, and photophobia. They are believed to be the result of intra-epithelial apical deposits in the cornea, conjunctiva, and lens epithelia [71]. Electron microscopy reveals these deposits to be lipid inclusion lamellar membranous bodies, similar to that observed in patients with Fabry's disease. The symptoms can usually be managed with artificial tears and generally resolve when the drug is discontinued.

A higher than expected incidence of severe and/or life-threatening infection has also been noted. This cannot be attributed to instrumentation with central venous catheters or internal urinary stents. Many of these infections have been documented in patients with normal granulocyte counts [66,72, 73,74]. Hypocalcemia, pericardial effusion, anaphylaxis, nausea, vomiting, urticaria, fever, proteinuria, rash, lymphopenia, and thrombocytopenia have also been reported [66,73].

Results of clinical investigations

The concept of the therapeutic window is based on phase I investigations at the National Cancer Institute. In studies of patients with primarily renal cell and adrenocortical carcinomas, no responses were observed below plasma concentrations of 200 μg/ml (140 μM), while toxicities were prohibitive above 300 μg/ml (208 μM). It is unclear, however, if the lower limit, 200 μg/ml, should be the same target concentration for different tumor types. Phase II trials are ongoing in several diseases [66]. This discussion, however, will focus on genitourinary malignancies.

Prostatic cancer

The rationale for investigating suramin in prostatic cancer includes 1) the observed growth-inhibitory effects of prostatic cancer cell lines in vitro and in vivo, 2) the known effects of suramin on growth-factor action, and 3) the adrenal inhibitory effects of the drug.

The initial trials at the NCI used the continuous infusion schedule described previously. Regression of soft-tissue masses was noted in 4 of 8 patients with measurable disease, and a decrease of 50% or greater in PSA in 7 of 11 (63%) patients with bone-only evaluable disease [75]. A confirmatory trial in patients with measurable disease at M.D. Anderson, the Mayo Clinic, and Memorial Sloan-Kettering Cancer Center was subsequently initiated. Of the first 17 evaluable patients, PR was noted in 1 (6%, 95% confidence limits 0–14%), and decreases in PSA (>50%) in 4 of 14 evaluable cases; accrual is continuing [73].

Subsequently, the NCI reported on 35 patients, 15 with measurable lesions, 21 with painful bony lesions, and 29 with baseline PSA >5x normal. Six of 15 (40%) had PR in measurable disease (three with no change in PSA), and 15 (70%) had an improvement in bone pain. Considering only PSA, 6 of 29 (21%) had a normalization, and 16 (55%) had a greater than 50% decrease from baseline. Median survivals were 9 months for those with soft tissue and 15 months for those with bone-only disease [76]. This is similar to a series of 146 patients treated with chemotherapy at MSKCC [77]. In order to eliminate a possible effect of the hydrocortisone, which has shown activity in patients with relapsed disease [78], a randomized trial of suramin plus hydrocortisone vs. hydrocortisone alone was organized. The trial was closed for lack of accrual.

The results in other centers have confirmed antitumor activity in hormone-refractory prostatic cancer. Ahmann et al. noted PR in 6 of 14 evaluable cases [74]. Three other studies focused primarily on PSA as the clinical trial endpoint. Regressions >50% were considered significant. A response was observed in 10 of 20 [79], 3 of 5 [80], and 4 of 9 [65] cases, respectively. In general, the duration of the response is generally short. It is unclear, however, if this reflects decreases in plasma concentrations or true progression. To confirm that suramin did not interfere with the Tandem-R PSA assay, we determined PSA in matched plasms samples with and without 250 μg/ml of suramin, and no differences were observed [81].

Adrenocortical carcinoma

Using a target concentration of 300 μg/ml, two partial and two minor responses were observed in 16 evaluable cases [19]. Five patients had stable disease for 3–10 months. The remainder progressed. Only one of the seven patients with abnormal secretion of steroid hormones had a documented decline in levels following suramin treatment. Median survivals were only 7 months [3].

Renal cell carcinoma

The rationale for an evaluation of suramin in renal cell carcinomas include the observation of increased expression of both EGF-r and TGF-alpha in the kidney, and that these factors are expressed at higher levels in renal cell cancer [82–85]. A heparin-binding growth factor similar to FGF has also been isolated [86]. This suggests a possible autocrine mechanism. Inhibition of renal cell carcinoma cell lines has been observed in vitro [87]. In addition, suramin is selectively concentrated in the kidney [68]. At the NCI, 1 of 3 patients treated in a phase I study showed PR radiographically with normalization of hypercalcemia, and one died from pneumonia with extensive tumor necrosis and no viable tumor at autopsy [19]. Clinical trials at the NCI and MSKCC have shown little activity [88,89].

Testicular cancer

Studies on the differentiation of the teratocarinoma cell line NTera-2 cl. D1 (NT2/D1) has shown that TGF-a and HST-1/kgf are downregulated after treatment with retinoic acid [90]. bFGF also declines. Subsequently it was shown that bFGF and HST-1/KFGF are coexpressed in $\frac{5}{7}$ nonseminoma and TGF-a in $\frac{4}{5}$ of the same cells [91]. These growth factors were found to stimulate cell growth in fetal calf serum but not in serum-free medium, suggesting that a combination of factors is important for cell growth and proliferation. This provides the rationale for phase II investigations in relapsed testicular tumors. A clinical trial is ongoing at MSKCC.

Bladder cancer

Although activity has been reported against bladder cancer cell lines in vitro, no clinical trials have been performed [92].

Future directions

Suramin represents the first of a class of putative growth factor inhibitors. The observed response proportions in patients with relapsed prostatic cancer, a disease for which no standard therapy exists, are encouraging. The short duration of response suggests the need to investigate schedules that maintain therapeutic concentrations for longer durations. It is not surprising considering that suramin is tumoristatic and not tumoricidal in many in vitro systems. In our studies with a continuous infusion schedule, a positive therapeutic effect correlated directly with total area under the concentration time curve, a measured time >100 μg/ml, and inversely, with the rate of elimination [87]. Using an intermittent parenteral dose schedule during the loading and maintenance phase, investigators at the University of Maryland maintained plasma concentrations in the range of 200–300 μg/ml until disease progression was documented. Dosing recommendations were adjusted using an adaptive control algorithm [73]. Preliminary data in nine patients showed decreases in prostate-specific antigen levels in eight (89%), with regression in soft-tissue disease in 3 of 3 cases [91]. The data suggest that flexible dosing can be used to target a given plasma concentration and that maintenance of plasma concentrations may maximize the chance of benefit [81,82].

While responses have been observed in renal cell carcinoma, where proliferation is also partially growth factor mediated, data are too preliminary to draw definitive conclusions. Studies in testicular cancer are continuing. The use of suramin is complex and the optimal dosing regimen has not been derived. Pharmacologic monitoring is essential, as there is a narrow therapeutic window. A key problem with suramin remains its lack of specificity, for, in addition to its growth-factor effects, it binds to a number of serum proteins, and inhibits lysosomal enzymes, protein kinase C, and glycolysis. A better understanding of the mechanism of action may allow more specific analogs to be developed.

The observed responses also suggest the need to investigating suramin in combination with chemotherapeutic and biologic agents. Preliminary data using prostate cancer cell lines suggest that synergistic effects, particularly with adriamycin and TNF, can be observed at relatively low ($<50\,\mu g/ml$) levels of suramin [41]. This may not only improve therapeutic outcome, but may also reduce toxicity. The minimal concertration to achieve antitumor efficacy is not known. Combinations with angiostatic steroids also warrant further study [93], as do studies on the inhibition of motility, a prerequisite for the development of metastatic disease [94]. Ultimately a better understanding of the biology of these tumors will improve the outcome. Isolating the active components of the GAGs generated by suramin may also permit the development of more specific inhibitors.

Acknowledgments

This work was supported by National Institutes of Health CA-05826 and CM-057732.

References

1. Albert A: *Selective Toxicity*. John Wiley and Sons, New York, 1965, pp. 68–98.
2. Hawking F: Suramin: With special reference to onchocerciasis. Adv Pharmacol Chemother 15:289–322, 1978.
3. La Rocca RV, Stein CY, Myers CE: Suramin: Prototype of a new generation of antitumor compounds. Cancer Cells 2:106–115, 1990.
4. Tobias N: Juvenile pemphigus: Treatment with Germanin (Bayer 205); report of a fatal case. Am J Dis Child 48:1084–1091, 1934.
5. Wells HG, Humphries EM, Work EG: Significance of the increased frequency of selective cortical necrosis of adrenal as a cause of Addison's disease. JAMA 109:490–493, 1937.
6. La Rocca RV, Stein CA, Danesi R, James-Dow CA, Weiss GH, Myers CE: Suramin in adrenal cancer: Modulation of steroid hormone production, cytotoxicity in vitro, and clinical antitumor effect. J Clin Endocrinol Metab 71:497–504, 1990.
7. De Clercq E: Suramin in the treatment of AIDS: Mechanism of action. Antiviral Res 7:1–10, 1987.

8. Cheson BD, Levine AM, Mildvan D, et al.: Suramin therapy in AIDS and related disorders. Report of the U.S. Suramin Working Group. JAMA 258:1347–1351, 1987.
9. Brody S, Collins JM, Markham PD, Relfield RR, Hoth DF, Groopman JE, Gallo RC, Yarchoan R, Lane HC, Klecker RW, Mitsuya H, Gelman E, Resnick L, Meyers CE, Fauci AS: Effects of suramin on HTLV-III/LAV infection presenting as Kaposi's sarcoma or AIDS related complex: Clinical pharmacology and suppression of virus replication in vivo. Lancet 2:627–630, 1985.
10. Collins JM, Klecker RW, Verchoan R, et al.: Clinical pharmacokinetics of suramin in patients with HTLV-III/LAV infection. J Clin Pharmacol 26:22–26, 1986.
11. Williams L, Tremble P, Lavin M, et al.: Platelet-derived growth factor receptors form a high affinity state in membrane preparations. J Biol Chem 259:5287–5294, 1984.
12. Hosang, M: Suramin binds to platelet-derived growth factor and inhibits its biologic activity. J Cell Biochem 29:265–273, 1985.
13. Ganelt JS, Coughlin JR, Niman HL, Tremble PM, Geils GM, Williams LT: Blockade of autocrine stimulation in simian sarcoma virus-transformed cells reverses down-regulation of platelet-derived growth factor receptors. Proc Natl Acad Sci USA 81:7466–7470, 1984.
14. Betsholtz C, Johnson A, Heldin C-H, Westermark B: Efficient reversion of simian sarcoma virus-trans-formation and inhibition of growth factor-induced mitogenesis by suramin. Proc Natl Acad Sci USA 83:6440–6444, 1986.
15. Huang SS, Huang JS: Rapid turnover of the platelet-derived growth factor receptor in sis-transformed cells and reversal by suramin. J Biol Chem 263:12608–12618, 1989.
16. Coffey RJ, Leof EB, Shipley GD, Moses HL: Suramin inhibition of growth factor receptor binding and mitogenicity in AKR-2B cells. J Cell Physiol 132:143–148, 1987.
17. Berns EMJJ, Schurmans ALG, Bolt J, et al.: Antiproliferative effects of suramin on androgen responsive tumour cells. Eur J Cancer 26:470–474, 1990.
18. Pollak M, Richard M: Suramin blockade of insulinlike growth factor I-stimulated proliferation of human osteosarcoma cells. J Natl Cancer Inst 82:1349–1352, 1990.
19. Stein CA, La Rocca RV, Thomas R, McAtee N, Myers CA: Suramin: An anticancer drug with a unique mechanism of action. J Clin Oncol 7:499–508, 1989.
20. Massague J: The TGF-b family of growth and differentiation factors. Cell 49:437–438, 1987.
21. Barnard JA, Lyons RM, Moses HL: The cell biology of transforming growth factor β. Biochem Biophys Acta 1032:79–97, 1990.
22. Wilding G, Zugmeier G, Knabbe C, Flanders K, Gelmann E: Differential effects of transforming growth factor b on human prostate cancer cells in vitro. Molec Cell Endocrinol 62:79087, 1989.
23. Shain SA, Lin AL, Koger JD, Karaganis AG: Rat prostate cancer cells contain functional receptors for transforming growth factor-b. Endrocrinology 126:818–825, 1990.
24. Rifkin DB, Moscatelli D: Recent developments in the cell biology of basic fibroblast growth factor. J Cell Biol 109:1–6, 1989.
25. Lyons RM, Moses HL: Transforming growth factors and the regulation of cell proliferation. Eur J Biochem 187:467–473, 1990.
26. Yayon A, Klagsbrun M: Autocrine transformation by chimeric signal peptide-basic fibroblast growth factor: Reversal by suramin. Proc Natl Acad Sci USA 87:5346–5350, 1990.
27. Moscatelli D, Quatro N: Transformation of NIH 3T3 cells with basic fibroblast growth factor or the hst/k-fgf oncogene causes down regulation of the fibroblast growth factor receptor: Reversal of morphological transformation and restoration of receptor number by suramin. J Cell Biol 109:2519–2527, 1989.
28. Roberts R, Gallagher J, Spooncer E, Allen TD, Bloofield F, Dexter TM: Heparan sulphate bound growth factors: A mechanism for stromal cell mediated haemopoiesis. Nature 332:376–378, 1988.
29. Thompson TC: Growth factors and oncogenes in prostatic cancer. Cancer Cells 2:345–354, 1990.
30. Connolly JM, Rose DP: Production of epidermal growth factor and transforming growth

factor alpha by the androgen-responsive LNCaP human prostate cancer cell line. The Prostate 16:209–218, 1990.
31. Wilding G, Valverius E, Knabbe C, Gelmann EP: Role of transforming growth factor alpha in human prostate cancer cell growth. The Prostate 15:1–12, 1989.
32. Mydlo JH, Bulbul MA, Richon VM, Heston WDW, Fair WR: Heparin-binding growth factor isolated from human prostatic extracts. The Prostate 12:343–355, 1988.
33. Mydlo JH, Michaeli J, Heston WDW, Fair WR: Expression of basic fibroblast growth factor mRNA in benign prostatic hyperplasia and prostatic carcinoma. The Prostate 13: 241–247, 1988.
34. Story MT, Sasse J, Jacobs SC, Lawson RK: Prostatic growth factor: Purification and structural relationship to basic fibroblast growth factor. Biochemistry 26:3843–3849, 1987.
35. Mansson PE, Adams P, Kan M, McKeehan WL: Heparin-binding growth factor gene expression and receptor characteristics in normal rat prostate and two transplantable rat prostate tumors. Cancer Res 49:2485–2494, 1989.
36. Mori H, Maki M, Oishi K, Jaye M, Igarashi K, Yoshida O, Hatanaka M: Increased expression of genes for fibroblast growth factor and transforming growth factor β-2 in human benign prostatic hyperplasia. The Prostate 13:241–247, 1990.
37. Hierowski MT, McDonald MW, Dunn L, Sullivan JW: The partial dependence of human prostatic growth factor on steroid hormones in stimulating thymidine incorporation into DNA. J Urol 138:909–912, 1987.
38. Nishi N, Matuo Y, Kuritomi K, Takenaka I, Usami M, Kotaki T, Wada F: The Prostate 13:39–48, 1988.
39. Horoszewicz JS, Leong SS, Kawinski E, Karr JP, Rosenthal TM, Chu TM, Mirand EA, Murphy GP: LNCaP model of human prostatic carcinoma. Cancer Res 43:1809–1818, 1983.
40. Lopes AD, Davis WL, Rosenstraus MJ, Uveques AJ, Gilman SC: Immunohistochemical and pharmacokinetic characterization of the site-specific immunoconjugate CYT-356 derived from antiprostate monoclonal antibody 7E11-C5. Cancer Res 50:6423–6429, 1990.
41. Freuhof JP, Myers CE, Sinha BK: Synergistic activity of suramin with tumor necrosis factor α and doxorubicin on human prostate cancer cell lines. J Natl Cancer Inst 82:1206–1209, 1990.
42. Martikainen P, Kyprianou N, Isaacs JT: Effect of transforming growth factor-β_1 on proliferation and death of rat prostatic cells. Endocrinology 127:2963–2968, 1990.
43. Ewing MW, LaRocca R, Stein CA, et al.: Effect of suramin on proliferation of human prostate carcinoma. Proc Am Assoc Cancer Res 30:310, 1989.
44. Rago R, Mitchen J, Cheng A, et al.: Metabolic effects of suramin (S) on human prostate cancer cells. Proc Am Assoc Cancer Res 31:1288, 1990.
45. Mitchen JL, Rago RP, Wilding G: Effects of suramin and TGFb on the proliferation of primary epithelial culture (PEC) for normal, benign hyperplastic (BPH) and cancerous human prostates. Proc Am Assoc Cancer Res 31:1289, 1990.
46. Morton RA, Isaacs JT, Isaacs WB: Differential effects of growth factor antagonists on neoplastic and normal prostatic cells. The Prostate 17:327–336, 1990.
47. Ono K, Nakare H, Fukushima M: Differential inhibition of various deoxyribonucleic and ribonucleic acid polymerases by suramin. Eur J Bichem 172:349–353, 1988.
48. Fortas PAG, Ellory JC, Lew JC: Suramin: A potent ATPase inhibitor which acts on the inside surface of the sodium pump. Biochem Biophys Acta 318:262–272, 1973.
49. Moriyana Y, Nelson N: Inhibition of vacuolar H^+-ATPases by fusidic acid and suramin. FEBS Lett 234:383–386, 1988.
50. Butler SJ, Kelly ECH, McKenzie FR, Guild SB, Wakelam MJO, Milligan G: Differential effects of suramin on the coupling of receptors to individual species of pertussis-toxin-sensitive guanine nucleotide-binding proteins. Biochem J 251:201–205, 1988.
51. Hensey CE, Boscoboinik D, Azzi A: Suramin, an anti-cancer drug, inhibits protein kinase C and induces differentiation in neuroblastoma cell clone NB2A. FEBS Lett 258:156–158, 1989.
52. Culouscou JM, Garrouste F, Remacle-Bonnet M, Bettetini D, Marvaldi J, Pommier G:

Autocrine secretion of a colorectum-derived growth factor by HT-29 human colon carcinoma cell line. Int J Cancer 42:895–901, 1988.
53. Fantini J, Rognoni J-B, Roccabianca M, Pommier G, Marvaldi J: Suramin inhibits cell growth and glycolytic activity and triggers differentiation of human colonic adenocarcinoma cell clone HT-29-D4. J Biol Chem 264:10282–10286, 1989.
54. Fantini J, Verrier B, Robert C, et al.: Suramin-induced differentiation of human colonic adenocarcinoma cell clone HT29-D4 in serum free medium. Exp Cell Res 89:109–17, 1990.
55. Davies M, Lloyd JB, Beck F: The effect of trypan blue, suramin and aurothiomalate on the breakdown of ^{125}I-labeled albumin within rat liver lysosomes. Biochem J 121:21–26, 1971.
56. Constantopoulos G, Rees S, Cragg BG, Barranger JA, Brady RO: Effect of suramin on the activities of degradative enzymes of sphingolipids in rats. Res Commun Chem Pathol Pharmacol 32:87–97, 1981.
57. Constantopoulos G, Rees S, Cragg BG, Barranger JA, Brady RO: Experimental animal model for mucopolysaccharidosis: Suramin induced glycosaminoglycan and sphingolipids accumulation in rat. Proc Natl Acad Sci USA 77:3700–3704, 1980.
58. Cooper MR, Danesi R, La Rocca R, Horne M, Myers CE: Suramin induces the production of anti-proliferative heparan sulfate in patients with malignancies (Abstr.). Proc Am Assoc Cancer Res 31:200, 1990.
59. Cooper M, La Rocca R, Stein C, Myers C: Pharmacokinetic monitoring is necessary for the safe use of suramin as an anticancer drug (Abstr.). Proc Am Assoc Cancer Res 30:242, 1989.
60. Klecker RW, Collins JM: Quantification of suramin by reverse-phase ion pairing high performance liquid chromatography. J Liquid Chromatogr 8:1685–1696, 1985.
61. Tong WP, Scher HI, Petrylak DP, Dnistrian A, Curley T, Vasquez J: A rapid assay of suramin in plasma. J Liquid Chromatogr 13:2269 2284, 1990.
62. Drusano GL, Forrest A, Snyder MJ, Reed MD, Blumer JL: An evaluation of optimal sampling strategy and adaptive study design. Clin Pharmacol Ther 44:232–238, 1988.
63. Forrest A, Scher HI, Tong W, Smart-Curley T, Vasquez J, Petrylak D: Development of an adaptive control algorithm for suramin (Abstr.). Proc Am Soc Clin Oncol 9:73, 1990.
64. Pinedo H, van Rijswijk Ren, Vu Academisch Ziekenhuis, Amsterdam, personal communication, 1990.
65. Van Oosterom At, De Simedt EA, Denis JJ, De Bruizn EA, Mahler C: Suramin for prostatic cancer: A phase I/II study in advanced extensively pretreated disease. Eur J Cancer 26:422, 1990.
66. Stein CA, LaRocca R, Myers C: Suramin: An old compound with new biology. Prin Pract Oncol 4:1–12, 1990.
67. LaRocca RV, Meer J, Gilliat RW, et al.: Suramin-induced polyneuropathy. Neurology 40:954–960, 1990.
68. Weiss GH, Jamis-Dow CA, Cooper MR, Linehan WM, Myers CE: Pharmacokinetics and biodistribution of suramin. J Urol 143:218(243A), 1990.
69. Eisan V, Loveday C: Effects of suramin on complement, blood clotting, fibrinolysis and kinin formation. Br J Pharmacol 49:678–687, 1973.
70. Horne MV, Stein CY, La Rocca RV, Myers CE: Circulating glycosaminoglycans anticoagulants associated with suramin treatment. Blood 71:273–279, 1988.
71. Holland EJ, Stein CA, Palestine AG, La Rocca RV, Chan CC, Kawabara T, Myers CE, Thomas R, McAtee T, Nussblatt RN: Suramin keratopathy. Am J Opthal 106:216–221, 1988.
72. Senderowicz A, Scher H, Gordon M, Petyrlak DP, Curley T, Motzer R, Bajorin DF: Infectious complications of suramin in patients with genitourinary tumors. Proc Am Assoc Cancer Res 32:(Abst 1213)203, 1991.
73. Christian M: T89–0084. Phase II trial of suramin in hormone refractory prostatic cancer. Personal communication.
74. Ahmann FR, Schwartz J, Dorr R, Salmon S: Suramin in hormone resistant metastatic prostate cancer: Significant anticancer activity but unanticipated toxicity. Proc Am Soc Clin Oncol 10:178(574), 1991.

75. Myers CE, Stein C, LaRocca R, Cooper M, Cassidy J, McAtee N: Suramin: An antagonist of heparin-binding tumor growth factors with activity against a broad spectrum of human tumors. Proc Am Soc Clin Oncol 8:66(256), 1989
76. Myers CE, LaRocca R, Stein C, Cooper M, Dawson N, Choyke P, Linehan M, Uhrich M: Treatment of hormonally refractory prostate cancer with suramin. Proc Am Soc Clin Onc 9:133(517), 1990.
77. Petrylak DP, Scher HI, Li, Z, Curley T, Geller N: Prognostic factors for survival of patients treated with single-agent chemotherapy bidimensionally measurable hormone refractory metastatic prostatic cancer (Abstr.). Proc Am Assoc Cancer Res 31:225, 1990.
78. Tannock I, Gospodarowicz M, Meakin W, Panzarella T, Stewart L, Rider W: Treatment of metastatic prostatic cancer with low-dose prednisone: Evaluation of pain and quality of life as pragmatic indices of response. J Clin Oncol 7:590–597, 1990.
79. Dawson N: Walter Reed Medical Center, personal communication, 1991.
80. Armand JP, Droz JP: Institute Gustave-Roussy, personal communication, 1991.
81. Scher HI, Nisselbaum J: Unpublished observations, 1990.
82. Nakamoto T, Usui A, Oshima K, et al.: Analysis of growth factors in renal cell carcinoma. Biochem Biophys Res Comm 153:818–824, 1988.
83. Mydlo J, Michaeli J, Cordon-Cardo C, et al.: Expression of transforming growth factor alpha and epidermal growth factor receptor messenger RNA in neoplastic and non-neoplastic human kidney tissue. Cancer Res 49:3407–3411, 1989.
84. Ambs KE, Takahashi A, Hering A, et al.: Epidermal growth factor receptor in adenocarcinoma of the kidney. Urol Res 17:251–254, 1989.
85. Sargent ER, Gomella L, Belldegrum A, et al.: Epidermal growth factor receptor gene expression in normal kidney and renal cell carcinoma. J Urol 142:1364–1368, 1989.
86. Rizzino A, Kuszynski C, Ruff E, Tiesman J: Production and utilization of growth factors related to fibroblast growth factor by embryonal carcinoma cells and their differentiated cells. Devel Biol 129:61–71, 1988.
87. Heston WDW, Fair WR, Huryk, R, Russo P: Growth inhibitory effect of suramin on urologic tumors in-vitro. 141:729(352A), 1989.
88. LaRocca RV, Stein CA, Danesi R, Cooper MR, Ulrich M, Myers CM. A pilot study of suramin in metastatic renal cell carcinoma. Cancer 67:1509–1513, 1991.
89. Iversen J, Scher H, Motzer R, Forrest A, Curley T, Tong W, Niedzwiecki D: Suramin (SUR): Impact of individualized pharmacokinetics (PK) dosing on outcome in patients with prostatic cancer (PC) and renal cell carcinoma (RCC). Proc Am Soc Clin Oncol 10:(Abst 103), 283, 1991.
90. Miller WH, May D, Li A, Gripp JF, Dmitrovsky E: Retinoic acid induces down-regulation of several growth factors and proto-oncogenes in a human embryonal cancer cell line. Oncogene, in press.
91. Dmitrovsky E, Moy D, Miller WH, Li A, Masui H: Retinoic acid causes a decline in cloning efficiency, tumorigenicity, and TGF-a expression in a human embryonal cancer cell line. Oncogene Res, in press.
92. Eisenberger M, Jodrell D, Sinibaldi V, Zuhowski E, Jacobs S, Egorin M, Van Echo DA: Preliminary evidence of anti-tumor activity against prostate cancer (PrCa) observed in a phase I trial with suramin. Proc Am Soc Clin Oncol 10: in press, 1991.
93. Wilks JW, DeKoning TF, Cocuzza JM, Tomilo A, Scott PS, Vrba LK: Suramin plus angiostatic steroids suppress tumor growth. Proc Am Assoc Cancer Res 31:60, 1990.
94. Pienta KJ, Coffey DS: Cancer cell motility as a chemotherapeutic target: Suramin and basic fibroblast growth factor. J Urol 143:214(242A), 1990.

Index

Acidic fibroblast growth factor (FGF), 135
Acrolein metabolites, MESNA therapy and, 13
Actinomycin D, *see* Dactinomycin
Adenocarcinomas, 77, 78
Adenosine triphosphatase (ATPase), suramin and, 140, 141
Adenosine triphosphate (ATP), suramin and, 140
Adrenal cortex toxicity, of suramin, 131, 137, 141, 142
Adrenalectomy, for prostatic cancer, 29
Adrenocortical carcinoma
  GU RMS and, 2
  suramin and, 144, 145
Adriamycin, *see* Doxorubicin
Afterloading technique, in brachytherapy, 67, 70
AIDS, suramin and, 131
Albumin, suramin and, 133–134, 141
Alcohol abuse, suramin and, 144
Alveolar rhabdomyosarcoma, 3, 4
Anandron, for prostatic cancer, 31–39
Anaphylaxis, suramin and, 144
Anaplastic carcinomas, 78
Anaplastic rhabdomyosarcoma, 4
Anastomotic malignancies, 75, 76, 77, 78, 79, 80
Androgen therapy, *see* Total androgen blockade
Anterior extenteration, for GU RMS, 13
Ascorbic acid, carcinogens and, 80
Autocrine growth factor production, 132, 134, 135, 137, 140, 146
Autotransplantation, in renal cell carcinoma, 21, 22

Bacillus Calmetter Guerin (BCG)
  for bladder cancer, 101, 102
  TNF and, 106
  for transitional cell carcinoma, 26
Bacterial endotoxin, TNF and, 106
Bacteriuria, uroenteric reconstructions and, 78, 82
Bartholin's gland infections, GU RMS mistaken for, 5
Basic fibroblast growth factor (b-FGF), 133, 134, 135, 146
Benign prostatic hypertrophy (BPH), suramin and, 136
Biopsies
  of GU RMS, 6, 13
  of prostatic cancer, 42, 44
  uroenteric reconstructions and, 82
Bladder augmentation
  GU RMS and, 10, 12
  malignancies associated with, 76
Bladder barbottage, uroenteric reconstructions and, 82
Bladder bilharziasis, uroenteric reconstructions and, 80
Bladder cancer
  neoadjuvant chemotherapy and cystectomy for, 99–103
  suramin for, 146
  TNF for, 116
  uroenteric reconstructions and, 80, 81
Bladder rhabdomyosarcoma, 1, 3, 4, 6, 7, 8, 9–10
Bladder salvage, in GU RMS, 8, 9, 12
Bleomycin, 90
Bone marrow aspiration, in GU RMS, 7, 13
Bone marrow metastases, in GU RMS, 2, 3
Bone marrow transplantation, in GU RMS, 15
Bone scans
  in GU RMS, 7, 13
  in prostatic cancer, 44
Bone surveys, in GU RMS, 7, 13
Botryoid rhabdomyosarcoma, 10
Brachytherapy, 65–73
  case selection in, 69
  clinical series in, 67–68
  description of, 67
  treatment planning in, 69–70
  treatment reactions in, 70–73

Brain tumors, 1, 2
Breast cancer, 2
Buserelin, for prostatic cancer, 32–39

Calcium, suramin and, 140
Carcinogens, uroenteric reconstructions and, 78, 79–80
Cathepsin, suramin and, 134
Cecocytoplasty, malignancies associated with, 76, 77
Cell motility, 121–129
  development of visual grading system for, 122–123
  preliminary studies of visual grading of, 126–128
  quantitative method of studying, 123–126
Central nervous system tumors, 2
Cervical rhabdomyosarcoma, 1, 8
Chemotherapy, *see also* specific agents
  for bladder cancer, 99–103
  for GU RMS, 3, 7, 8–9, 10, 11–12, 13, 14
  intravesical, 116
  for prostatic cancer, 60
  for testicular cancer, 89, 90, 91, 96
  for transitional cell carcinoma, 25, 26
Chondroitan sulfate, suramin and, 144
Cisplatin
  for GU RMS, 11
  TNF and, 111
C-myc oncogene, GU RMS and, 3
Collagenase IV activity, suramin and, 134
Colocytoplasty, malignancies associated with, 76, 77
Colon carcinoma, 75, 80, 81, 82
Colon conduits, malignancies associated with, 78
Colonoscopy, in uroenteric reconstructions, 76
Colostomy, radiation therapy and, 48
Computed tomography (CT)
  in bladder cancer, 100
  in GU RMS, 6, 7, 13, 14
  in prostatic cancer, 42
  in testicular cancer, 92
  in transitional cell carcinoma, 25
Cyclophosphamide, 8–9, 13, 14, *see also* VAC therapy
Cyproterone acetate, for prostatic cancer, 30
Cystectomy
  for bladder cancer, 99–103
  for GU RMS, 9–10, 12
  for transitional cell carcinoma, 25
Cystography, in uroenteric reconstructions, 82
Cystoplasty, malignancies associated with, 82
Cystoprostatectomy, for GU RMS, 12
Cytogenetics, of GU RMS, 2
Cytologic examinations
  of transitional cell carcinoma, 25
  of uroenteric reconstructions, 82
Cytomorphometry, static, 53
Cytoscopy, in GU RMS, 6
Cytotoxicity
  of suramin, 140
  of TNF, 107, 108, 111

Dactinomycin (Actinomycin D), *see also* VAC therapy; VAI therapy
  for GU RMS, 7, 8–9, 11, 12
  TNF and, 105, 107, 108, 111, 112, 113
Dermatan sulfate, suramin and, 141
Desquamation, radiation therapy and, 48
Dexamethasone, 138
Dialysis, transitional cell carcinoma and, 25
Diarrhea, radiation therapy and, 48
Dicarbazine (DTIC), 11
Diethylstilbesterol (DES), 136–137
α-Difluormethylornithine, 81
Digital rectal examination, 41, 44
Dihydrotestosterone (DHT), 137–138
Dizziness, TAB and, 36
DNA
  carcinogens and, 79
  GU RMS and, 2, 3
  suramin and, 133
  TNF and, 113–115
DNA aneuploid tumors
  in GU RMS, 3
  in prostatic cancer, 53, 54, 55, 56, 57, 58, 60
DNA diploid tumors, in prostatic cancer, 53, 54, 55, 56, 57, 58–60
DNA ploidy
  in GU RMS, 3
  in prostatic cancer, 53–60
DNA tetraploid tumors, in prostatic cancer, 53, 54, 56, 57, 58, 60
DNA topoisomerase II-targeted drugs, *see* Topoisomerase II-targeted drugs
Doxorubicin (Adriamycin)
  for GU RMS, 8, 11
  suramin and, 147
  TNF and, 111, 112, 115, 117
  topoisomerase II and, 109
DynaCELL, 124
Dysplasia, uroenteric reconstructions and, 82
Dysuria, radiation therapy and, 48

EGF, *see* Epidermal growth factor
EGFR oncogene, GU RMS and, 3
Ejaculation, RPLND and, 91, 92, 96
Electroresection, for transitional cell carcinoma, 26
Embryonal rhabdomyosarcoma, 3–4, 10, 13, 14

Endoscopy, in uroenteric reconstructions, 82
Endosomes, suramin and, 141
Endothelial cells, suramin and, 134, 136
Enterocytoplasty, malignancies associated with, 75, 76–78
Epidermal growth factor (EGF)
  suramin and, 133–134, 145
  uroenteric reconstructions and, 81
Epithelial cells, suramin and, 134, 138, 139
Estrogen therapy, for prostatic cancer, 29, 53
Etoposide (VP-16), *see also* VIE therapy
  for GU RMS, 11, 12
  for testicular cancer, 90
  TNF and, 111, 112, 113, 115, 117
  topoisomerase II and, 109
Eulexin (Flutamide), 30
Extracorporeal surgery, for renal cell carcinoma, 21–22

Fabry's disease, 144
Fecal incontinence, radiation therapy and, 48
Fertility
  GU RMS and, 14
  RPLND and, 90, 92
Fetal alcohol syndrome, 2
α-Fetoprotein, 92
Fever, suramin and, 144
FGF, *see* Fibroblast growth factor
Fibrinogen, suramin and, 141
Fibroblast growth factor (FGF), 131, 133, 134–136, 143, 145, 146
  acidic, 135
  basic, 133, 134, 135, 146
Fibroblasts, growth factors and, 136
Fibronectin receptors, suramin and, 134
Fibroplasia, b-FGF and, 134
Fibrosarcomas, 107
Fibrosis
  radiation therapy and, 67
  RPLND and, 91
Flow cytometry
  in GU RMS, 3
  in prostatic cancer, 53–54, 55–56, 57, 60
Fluorouracil, 111
Flutamide (Eulexin), 30
Fourier analysis, of cell motility, 124–126

Genitourinary rhabdomyosarcoma (GU RMS), 1–15
  clinical presentation of, 4–5
  cytogenetics of, 2
  diagnosis of, 6
  epidemiology of, 1–2
  molecular studies of, 2–3
  pathology of, 3–4
  prognosis in, 10–13
  radiographic evaluation of, 5–6
  treatment of, 7–10
gli oncogene, GU RMS and, 2
Globulins, suramin and, 141
Glucocorticoids, 138
β-Glucuronidase, suramin and, 141
Glycolysis, suramin and, 147
Glycosoaminoglycans (GAGs), suramin and, 141, 143, 144, 147
Gorlin's basal-cell nevus syndrome, 2
G proteins, suramin and, 140
Grading
  of prostatic cancer, 53, 54, 121–129
  of renal cell carcinoma, 20
  of transitional cell carcinoma, 25, 26
Granulocyte macrophage colony stimulating factor (GM-CSF), 135
Growth factor antagonists, suramin in development of, 131–147, *see also* Suramin
Guanosine triphosphatase (GTPase), suramin and, 140
Guillain-Barre syndrome, suramin and, 143
GU RMS, *see* Genitourinary rhabdomyosarcoma

Headaches, TAB and, 36
Heparan, suramin and, 141, 144
Heparan sulfate proteoglycans, suramin and, 135
Heparin, 24
  FGF and, 134
Heparin-binding growth factors, 135, 136, 145–146
Hot flashes, TAB/testicular ablation and, 36
hst/K-fgf oncogene, suramin and, 135, 146
hst-1/kgf oncogene, suramin and, 146
β-Human chorionic gonadotrophin (HCG), 92
Hyaluronidase, suramin and, 141
Hydrocortisone, suramin and, 142, 145
Hypercalcemia, suramin and, 146
Hyperfractionated radiation therapy, for GU RMS, 12
Hypocalcemia, suramin and, 144
Hypophysectomy, for prostatic cancer, 29
Hysterectomy, for GU RMS, 7, 11, 12–13

Iduronate sulfatase, suramin and, 141
Iduronate synthetase, suramin and, 141
Ifosfamide, 12, 13
Ileal conduit urinary diversion, malignancies associated with, 78
Ileocytoplasty, malignancies associated with, 76, 77
Impotence, TAB/testicular ablation and, 36
Insulin, 137
Interferons, 105
Interleukin-2 (IL-2), 105, 116

Interstitial pneumonitis, TAB and, 36, 38
Intravenous pyelography (IVP)
  in GU RMS, 5–6
  in transitional cell carcinoma, 25
Intravenous urography, in uroenteric reconstructions, 82
Intravesical chemotherapy, 116
Intravesical tumor necrosis factor (TNF), 116
Iodine-125 implants, 57
Iridium-192 implants, 67, 68, 70, 73

Jackson staging system, 65, 68

Kaposi's sarcoma, suramin and, 131
Keratopathy, suramin and, 144
Kidneys, suramin concentration in, 146
Kupffer cells, suramin and, 143

Laparoscopy, in prostatic cancer, 43
Laparotomy, for GU RMS, 6
Laser fulgeration, for transitional cell carcinoma, 26
Leuprolide, 30
LHRH, *see* Luteinizing hormone releasing hormone
Libido loss, TAB/testicular ablation and, 36
Liver toxicity, of suramin, 143–144
L-myc oncogene, GU RMS and, 3
Lung cancer, 111
Lung metastases, in GU RMS, 3
Lupron, 30
Luteinizing hormone-releasing hormone (LHRH)
  DNA ploidy and, 58, 60
  in testicular ablation, 30, 31, 32–39
Lymphadenectomy, 44, 48, 49, 57, *see also* Retroperitoneal lymph-node dissections
Lymphangiography, in GU RMS, 14
Lymphatic metastases, in GU RMS, 3, 4, 5
Lymphocytes, TNF and, 116
Lymphoid cells, suramin and, 134
Lymphopenia, suramin and, 144
Lysosomes, suramin and, 141, 143, 147

Macrophages, carcinogens and, 81
Magnetic resonance imaging (MRI)
  in GU RMS, 6
  in prostatic cancer, 42, 43
Major histocompatibility complex (MHC), 106
Mastectomy, 66
Mesenchymal cells
  GU RMS and, 3
  suramin and, 134, 135
MESNA therapy, 13
Metastases
  in bladder cancer, 99
  bone marrow, 2, 3
  in GU RMS, 2, 3, 4, 5, 7, 8, 10, 12, 13, 15
  lung, 3
  lymphatic, 3, 4, 5
  in prostatic cancer, 44–45, 121–129
  in testicular cancer, 89
Methotrexate, 111, *see also* M-VAC therapy
Mitomycin C, 26
Molecular studies, of GU RMS, 2–3
Monoclonal antibodies, GU RMS and, 3
Monomorphous round-cell rhabdomyosarcoma, 4
mRNA
  dactinomycin and, 108
  gli, 2
  topoisomerase II and, 109
Mucopolysaccharidosis, suramin and, 141
M-VAC therapy
  for bladder cancer, 99–103
  for transitional cell carcinoma, 26
Myeloid cells, suramin and, 134

Nausea
  suramin and, 144
  TAB and, 36
Necrosis
  brachytherapy and, 73
  testicular cancer and, 90, 91
Neoadjuvant chemotherapy, cystectomy and, 99–103
Neovascularization, b-FGF and, 134
Nephrectomy
  for renal cell carcinoma, 20, 21, 22, 24
  for transitional cell carcinoma, 25
Nephrogenic adenomas, 78
Nephroscopy, in transitional cell carcinoma, 26
Nephroureterectomy, for transitional cell carcinoma, 25
NEU oncogene, GU RMS and, 3
Neuroblastomas, 1
Neurofibromatosis, 2
Nitrates, 80, 81
Nitrites, 80, 81
Nitrosamines, 80, 81
N-Nitroso compounds, 79–80, 82–83
Nitrosourea methyl-CCNU, 2
N-myc oncogene, GU RMS and, 3
Nonseminomatous germ cell tumor, testicular, 89–96
N-ras oncogene, GU RMS and, 2
Nuclear DNA ploidy, *see* DNA ploidy
Nulutimide, *see* Anandron

Oat cell carcinomas, 77
Orchiectomy, *see also* Testicular ablation
  for GU RMS, 13
  for testicular cancer, 92, 96
Ornithine decarboxylase, 81

Osteoblasts, growth factors and, 136
Ovarian carcinoma, 116

Pain
in prostatic cancer, 33, 38
radiation therapy and, 48
Paracrine growth factor production, 134, 137
Paratesticular rhabdomyosarcoma, 1, 3, 13–15
Paris system of dosimetry, 70
PDGF, *see* Platelet-derived growth factor
Pelvic extenteration, for GU RMS, 7, 11
Pemphigus, 131
Penectomy, 66, 68, 73
Penile carcinoma, 65–73
epidemilogy and pathobiology of, 65
staging of, 65–66, 68
Pericardial effusion, suramin and, 144
Photophobia, suramin and, 144
Plasminogen activators, FGF as, 135
Platelet-derived growth factor (PDGF), 132–133, 134, 135
Pleomorphic rhabdomyosarcoma, 3, 4
Polymerases, suramin and, 131, 140
Polypectomy, for GU RMS, 11
Polypoid tumors
in GU RMS, 12
uroenteric reconstructions and, 79, 82
Polyps, uroenteric reconstructions and, 76
Polyradiculopathy, suramin and, 143
Prostatectomy, 12
DNA ploidy and, 55, 56, 57, 58
radiation therapy following, 41–49
Prostate-specific antigen (PSA)
DNA ploidy and, 58–60
prostatectomy and, 42–43, 44, 45
radiation therapy and, 48, 49
suramin and, 137, 145
Prostatic acid phosphatase, 33, 137
Prostatic cancer
cell motility in, 121–129
DNA ploidy and, 53–60
mortality from, 34–35, 38–39
pain in, 33, 38
radiation therapy following prostatectomy for, 41–49
suramin for, 135–139, 142, 144–145, 147
TAB vs. testicular ablation for, 29–39
Prostatic rhabdomyosarcoma, 1, 3, 4–5, 7, 8, 10
Proteinases, suramin and, 134
Protein kinase C, suramin and, 147
Proteinuria, suramin and, 144
Prothrombin, suramin and, 144
Pruritus, TAB and, 36
PSA, *see* Prostate-specific antigen
Pyeloscopy, in transitional cell carcinoma, 26

Radiation therapy, 60, *see also* Brachytherapy
for GU RMS, 7, 8, 9, 12, 13, 14
hyperfractionated, 12
as prostatectomy adjuvant, 41–49
Radiographic evaluation, of GU RMS, 5–6
Radionuclide bone scans, *see* Bone scans
Radium-226 implants, 67
Radium molds, 66–67
Rashes, suramin and, 144
5 α-Reductase, in prostatic cancer, 60
Renal cell carcinoma
renal-sparing surgery for, 19–24
suramin for, 144, 145–146, 147
TNF for, 113
Renal-sparing surgery, 19–26
for renal cell carcinoma, 19–24
for transitional cell carcinoma, 24–26
Retinoic acid, suramin and, 146
Retrograde pyelography, in transitional cell carcinoma, 25
Retroperitoneal lymph-node dissection (RPLND), 89–96
ejaculation and, 91, 92, 96
fertility and, 90, 92
in GU RMS, 13–14
nerve-sparing techniques in, 90, 91–96
RNA reverse transcriptase, suramin and, 131
RPLND, *see* Retroperitoneal lymph-node dissection

Sarcoma botryoides, 4
Schwann cells, suramin and, 143
Seizures, chemotherapy and, 13
Selenium, suramin and, 137
Side effects, *see also* specific side effects
of radiation therapy, 48–49
of TAB/testicular ablation, 36, 39
Simian sarcoma virus, suramin and, 132
sis cells, suramin and, 132, 133
Sphingoid hydrolases, suramin and, 141
Squamous cell carcinoma, 111
Staging
cell motility in, 127
of GU RMS, 7
of penile carcinoma, 65–66, 68
of prostatic cancer, 42–43, 44, 53, 127
of renal cell carcinoma, 20
of testicular cancer, 90, 92
of transitional cell carcinoma, 25
Static cytomorphometry, for prostatic cancer, 53
Steroid hormones, 30, *see also* specific types
suramin and, 131, 145
Suicide, penectomy and, 66
Superoxides, 81
Suramin, 131–147
action mechanisms of, 132–135

non-growth factor activities of, 140–141
pharmacology of, 141–143
for prostatic cancer, 135–139, 142, 144–145, 147
toxicity of, *see* under Toxicity
Surgery, 3, 7, 8, 9, *see also* specific types

TAB, *see* Total androgen blockade
Telangiectasia, radiation therapy and, 67
Teratoma, in testicular cancer, 89, 91
Testicular ablation, for prostatic cancer, 29–39
mortality rates and, 34–35, 38–39
response to, 34
side effects of, 36, 39
Testicular cancer
RPLND for, 89–96
suramin for, 146, 147
TGF, *see* Transforming growth factor
Thiotepa, 26
Thrombocytopenia
suramin and, 144
TNF and, 115
Time-lapse videomicroscopy, of cell motility, 121, 122, 124, 127
TNF, *see* Tumor necrosis factor
TNM classification system, 65–66
Topoisomerase II-targeted drugs, 105–117, *see also* specific agents
in vitro effects of, 110–111
in vivo effects of, 112–113
Total androgen blockade (TAB), for prostatic cancer, 29–39
mortality rates and, 34–35, 38–39
response to, 34
side effects of, 36, 39
Toxicity
adrenal cortex, 131, 137, 141, 142
cellular, *see* Cytotoxicity
liver, 143–144
of suramin, 131, 137, 141, 142, 143–144, 147
of TNF, 105, 115, 116
Transferrin, suramin and, 137
Transforming growth factor (TGF)
GU RMS and, 2
suramin and, 133, 134, 135, 138, 145, 146
Transforming growth factor-alpha (TGF-α), 135, 145, 146
Transforming growth factor-beta (TGF-β), 133, 134, 135, 138
Transitional cell carcinoma
renal-sparing surgery for, 24–26
uroenteric reconstructions and, 77
Trypanosomiasis, 131
Trypan red dye, 131
Tuberculosis, uroenteric reconstructions and, 76
Tubulin, GU RMS and, 2
Tumor cell inhibitory factors, GU RMS and, 2
Tumor enucleation, for renal cell carcinoma, 20, 21, 22–23
Tumor grading, *see* Grading
Tumor-infiltrating lymphocytes (TIL), TNF and, 116
Tumor necrosis factor (TNF), 105–117
anticancer effects of, 106–107
intravesical, 116
suramin and, 137, 138, 147
synergistic effects of, 113–115
in vitro effects of, 110–111
in vivo effects of, 112–113
Tumor staging, *see* Staging

Ultrasound
in GU RMS, 5, 14
in prostatic cancer, 42, 43, 44
in uroenteric reconstructions, 82
Undifferentiated sarcomas, 77
Ureteral reimplantation, in GU RMS, 12
Ureterosigmoidostomy, malignancies associated with, 75, 76, 78, 79, 80, 81, 82
Urethral salvage, in GU RMS, 12
Urethral stenosis, brachytherapy and, 68
Urinary diversion
malignancies associated with, 75, 78
radiation therapy and, 48
Urinary incontinence, radiation therapy and, 48
Urinary tract infections, uroenteric reconstructions and, 78, 80
Urinary tract reconstructions, *see* Uroenteric reconstructions
Uroenteric reconstructions, 75–83
clinical data on, 75–78
patient surveillance and, 81–82
tumor pathogenesis and, 79–81
Urticaria, suramin and, 144
Uteral reimplantation, GU RMS and, 10
Uterine rhabdomyosarcoma, 1, 5, 6, 8, 11
Uteropyeloscopy, in transitional cell carcinoma, 25
Uteroscopy, in transitional cell carcinoma, 25

VAC therapy, 8–9, 11, 12, *see also* M-VAC therapy
Vaginal rhabdomyosarcoma, 1, 5, 6, 7, 8, 11, 12–13
Vaginectomy, for GU RMS, 9, 11, 13
VAI therapy, 12
VA therapy, 8, 11
Vesicosigmoidostomy, malignancies associated with, 79, 81
VIA therapy, 14
Videomicroscopy, *see* Time-lapse

videomicroscopy
VIE therapy, 12
Vincristine, 2, 8–9, 12, 13, *see also* VAC therapy
Viremia, suramin and, 131
Vision problems
suramin and, 144
TAB and, 36
Vomiting
suramin and, 144
TAB and, 36
VP-16, *see* Etoposide
Vulvar rhabdomyosarcoma, 1, 5

Wilm's tumor, 1

X-ray therapy, 66, 67

Zoladex, for prostatic cancer, 30